PRAISE FOR

MAKING OUT LIKE A VIRGIN
Sex, Desire & Intimacy After Sexual Trauma

"This collection fills a gap in available literature ... a gift for those of us working alongside survivors and those of us who are survivors ourselves." *Jen Friedlander, Washington Coalition of Sexual Assault Programs*

"Through these powerful, beautiful stories we recognize that life is complicated, messy, painful, and damaging. But like the phoenix from the ashes, healing hope, driving passions, and a deep love of self can be born amidst the rubble. What a sweet and inspiring gift to receive: Stories that promise a life beyond the trauma – one that is vibrant, passionate, and full of possibility." *Auburn L. Watersong, Associate Director of Public Policy, Vermont Network Against Domestic and Sexual Violence and Episcopal priest*

"What a gift to anyone recovering from sexual trauma or anyone wanting to accompany them on their journeys to recovery and fulfillment." *David Walsh, Ph.D. Psychologist and author of* Why Do They Act That Way? A Survival Guide to the Adolescent Brain for You and Your Teen

"Rich in honest details, these stories are compelling reading." *Cheryl Burghdorf, Professor of English, retired*

"I wish I had read the book with a highlighter in hand so that I could create the mosaic within it that is 'my story.' More than that, I bless all of the story tellers and collectors for presenting the first book about child sexual assault that has ever made me feel understood, heard, accepted into a community, and healthy in my recovery. The telling of our stories is not only part of personal healing but, I hope, a part of a global healing that must begin." *Yehudit Zicklin-Sidikman, International Empowerment Self-defense Advocate and CEO/Co-founder El HaLev NGO*

"As a faculty member who teaches mostly young college women and those with sexual and gender minority identities, not a semester goes by without at least one student telling me of a recent experience of sexual trauma and all too many sharing histories of trauma and abuse. Some ask me if they will ever 'recover' and be able to reclaim their full selves. I tell them it is a long, slow, non-linear process, but yes, I believe it is possible. With the publication of this book, my students will no longer have to take my word for this!" *Jacqueline S. Weinstock, Ph.D., Human Development & Family Studies, University of Vermont*

"These stunning essays of courage and transcendence remind us that the human soul is mighty, and that love is always possible. They will make you weep with joy." *Karin Anderson, Honorary Board Member, Planned Parenthood of Northern New England and former Maine Women's Fund Executive Director*

"Unlike other stories by survivors, these have been fully processed, some beautifully written, all self-reflective and showing insight uncommon to victimization narratives…. Immensely helpful to those who call themselves victims and those who call themselves survivors and those readers looking for a more complex understanding of sexuality after trauma, growth, recovery, and healing." *Sharon Lamb, Ed.D., Ph.D., ABPP, winner of the Books for a Better Life Award, for* Packaging Girlhood, *and the Society for Sex Therapy and Research's Book Award for* Sex, Therapy, and Kids

"As a senior program officer who has been working to change the cultural acceptance of violence against women and children, I can't say enough about how important the stories are. Their tales of resilience offer hope to others who have been traumatized, to those who work in the helping/healing field, and to those of us who envision a world in which the forces of light have prevailed." *Karen Heck, Senior Program Officer, The Bingham Program, Tufts Medical Center*

"A poignant, diverse and courageous collection of experiences of sexual trauma that celebrate our resilience as human beings to survive, heal, and live full and satisfying lives." *Maine Coalition Against Sexual Assault*

"Finally, a book that explores the effects of sexual assault on both women and men. Understanding that sexual assault is a systemic problem and tackling it on an individual, community, family, and societal level are essential to the elimination of sexual assault as an acceptable norm in our communities and societies. But until then, survivors can hear from other survivors that healing is attainable. Thank you for writing this book, and readers and Freedom Fighters, thank you for reading it." *Wendi Dragonfire, Founder, Shuri-Ryu and Empowerment Self Defense, Netherlands and Germany*

"An essential book about sexual trauma that chronicles the many ways that people move forward." *Luca Maurer, program director and co-author of The Teaching Transgender Toolkit*

"After 26 years of working with well over 800 male survivors and a couple dozen female survivors, I am well aware of the range of losses (or thefts) experienced by survivors of sexual abuse. However, the greatest theft is the loss of true intimacy—emotional, psychological, or sexual. The testimonies offer specific examples of the real possibility of regaining one's natural, joyful, and fulfilling sexual and emotional connectedness. It's not just a lovely sounding theory, this book gives concrete examples and thereby a newfound hope." *Don Wright M.Ed., Founder/Executive Director, BC. Society for Male Survivors of Sexual Abuse, Vancouver, BC, Canada*

MAKING OUT LIKE A VIRGIN

Sex, Desire & Intimacy After Sexual Trauma

Edited by Catriona McHardy and Cathy Plourde

PORTLYN MEDIA

ANIMAL MINERAL PRESS, LLC

MAKING OUT LIKE A VIRGIN
Sex, Desire & Intimacy After Sexual Trauma
FIRST EDITION

Interior design by K. Larson
Cover design by kd diamond
Printed in the United States of America.

Library of Congress Control Number: 2016946721
ISBN-10: 1-944568-00-X
ISBN-13: 978-1-944568-00-9

PORTLYN MEDIA
AN IMPRINT OF ANIMAL MINERAL PRESS, LLC

Animal Mineral Press books may be purchased for educational, business, or sales promotional use. For information please write: Animal Mineral Press, Special Markets: animalmineralpress@gmail.com

We dedicate this book to those who have experienced sexual trauma in their lives. We hope in due time they will find a way out from under the labels of victim and survivor to meet themselves as they wish to be in the world, open to all of the sex, lust, and intimacy they desire.

For the coming generations, with optimism and hope for you: Tracy, Jennifer, Isabella, Megan, Catriona, Nathaniel, Tim, and Matt. And to Dee, whose arms will always keep me believing.
~C.M

K.L., you are the reason.
Each kiss a heart-quake... Lord Byron
~C.P.

What of soul was left, I wonder,
when the kissing had to stop?

Robert Browning

I'm on the hunt for who I've not yet become.

Sara Bareilles

CONTENTS

FOREWORD

Can those who have experienced sexual abuse really "make out like a virgin?"

Yes; with luck and courage.

What ties together these extraordinary stories of sexual re-birth is the willingness to start over, to invite another person to touch your emotional scars. The stakes involved in these acts of love are much higher than for that first kiss, that first undressing. This is a more revelatory, a more complete nakedness, as these sexual moments are as much about one's soul as about sex. This openness to emotional intimacy is, in many ways, how survivors of trauma feel like virgins—by encountering an altogether new way to engage in sex—one that's emotional as well as physical.

Sex is never just about sex. As these pages make abundantly clear, sex can be about power, comfort, domination, awareness, discovery, tenderness, violence, and identity. And that's the short list. The sexual relations that we undertake with each other—sometimes, unfortunately, under coercion that is physical, mental, or emotional—embody a deep, existential dynamic between humans. In the best of circumstances we open our arms and our psyches to someone else in the hope, the expectation, that our vulnerability will be reciprocated, and in that process we will be made whole. In the less-than-best of circumstances this path toward wholeness, already fraught with peril, becomes genuinely terrifying. One reason why this book is of utmost importance is that the authors in these pages guide us through these fears and toward the ultimate joy of a fulfilling sexual journey.

My own life has been shaped by someone else's mis-love of me. As an incest survivor, I spent a part of my adult life confusing sex with love, a destructive lesson taught to me, as a child, by my father. As an adult I struggled with a sexual addiction. In short, addiction is a common response, often repeated, when someone experiences sex in a context outside of love. As an adult, I was looking for love—as that country-and-western song says—in all the wrong places. And with all the wrong, emotionally dangerous men.

Another pattern that becomes clear in *Making Out Like a Virgin* is the importance of finding someone who can listen, empathize, understand. For me, this was a therapist who specialized in sexual addiction recovery. He non-judgmentally understood my struggle and helped me untangle those threads of sex and love. I had individual therapy sessions with him, but an even more important part of my learning the emotional relationship between sex and love took place in group therapy. There, I felt a part of something greater than myself; I felt deeply connected to people with similar experiences. We struggled to overcome our pasts together.

Similarly, beyond the power of each individual revelation in *Making Out Like a Virgin* is the collective power of a community of people who have refused to let the circumstances of their younger selves dictate the course of the rest of their lives. The individuals in this community have found the strength to become sexually and emotionally whole—a healing that transcends gender and orientation. The beauty of this book is that we, as readers, are given the opportunity to delve into the lives of people who are extraordinary by virtue of their refusal to have their sexual lives taken away from them. This does not mean that their lives have not been changed. They have. But by refusing to have one entire aspect of life obliterated, they collectively show that the lines that divide us are not those of male/female/trans/non-binary, heterosexual/gay/questioning, but those of abuser and survivor. The real division is between those who possess grace, and those who are graceless.

These are stories of grace. Not grace easily discovered, but one that evolves from internal struggle. This is the grace of doing whatever it takes to be a complete, authentic person. The authors of these essays could have lived lives that were partial and incomplete, thus shutting themselves off from others. It is fitting that these writers have come together in an anthology. This is yet another way in which they have overcome the isolation that could have resulted from the abuse they endured had it not been for their willingness to let sex become positive and, for some, even a spiritual force in their lives.

If you, too, have experienced abuse, here you will find that there are myriad paths to healing and fulfillment. Because the grace of these writers really *is* hard-won, you will discover that it is all right to have times when you feel alone, will discover that it is all right to sometimes *want* to be alone. As one writer puts it, "it's not all sunshine, rainbows, and lollipops." If you haven't experienced abuse, you'll find that stereotypes don't apply. Abuse transcends gender, class, race, and culture. So does survival.

This is an important and vital collection of voices. While the individual circumstances of these authors vary widely, the one thing they all have in common is their refusal to remain silent. These are voices that are empowering, urgent and, yes, sexy.

Sue William Silverman, author,
Love Sick: One Woman's Journey through Sexual Addiction

A Kiss is Just a Kiss

They say a kiss is just a kiss.

In reality, a kiss is the beginning of that joyful feeling of sexual arousal, when desire and excitement soar, where we lose ourselves and want the kiss to go on forever. Bodies move closer, caught up in the pleasure of touching of genitals, breasts, the nape of the neck. Lust wants in. The feeling of primal intimacy allows that lust to blossom, electrifying skin, and opening one's mind to erotic desire.

Imagine making out for the first time and the intensity of never having done it before. You want to do it because it is exciting, pure, and yes, a *virginal* experience.

Sexual expression is a natural part of who we are. We all want to enjoy and like our bodies, to desire and be desired, to experience sexual pleasure and the intimate feeling of trust and letting go. We want the inherent, vital, and often elusive essence of being sexually alive.

And yet, countless among us are denied this pleasure. Sexuality is so often hidden behind shyness, insecurity, and secrecy. Insecurity heightens the existing norms of a society fearful of natural human instincts. Disparities regarding sexual expression can debilitate us. Pervasive acts of sexual violence rob us of our ability to feel sexually healthy, resulting in personal devastation and an inablity to successfully navigate life, relationships, and career. These acts of violence fall on a continuum of behaviors — from threat of harm to threat fulfilled, from recurring verbal assault to rape.

Collectively, we have much work to do to eradicate sexual abuse and trauma, which hinders the lives of girls, boys, women, men and those overriding the binary boundaries of maleness and femaleness — whether the violence was a one-time, life-changing horror; years of injury; or part of a considered, systemic tool for oppression. People struggling with the after-effects of sexual assault and domestic violence can be found in staggering numbers around the world. The scars and wounds remain while cultural norms continue to keep everyday injustices and past memories alive. The systems that are supposed to protect and serve often operate in ways that further traumatize, even stigmatize, the individual and discourage others from coming forward.

We ask:

Why aren't institutions and their policies committed to helping survivors of sexual trauma reach full recovery?

What if children were taught their bodies are their own?

Why aren't men and boys acknowledged as victims and survivors of widespread abuse?

What if people understood that "the rules" of marriage or commitment do not always have to be forever?

What if boys and young men weren't taught and pressured to prove their masculinity?

What if there were adequately funded, evidence-based, long-term programs to rehabilitate offenders?

What if parents and teens accepted that sexual desire is a healthy part of adolescent development?

What if national attention was given to the well-documented fact that child abuse has long-term health effects, including fatality?

What if all social dictates surrounding gender expectations and roles were exposed and examined?

Again: *Why aren't institutions and their policies committed to helping survivors of sexual trauma reach full recovery?*

We need to find answers and explore solutions that serve a diversity of people and experiences regardless of age, race, ability, resources, gender, ethnicity, and geography. Vigilant, courageous champions have been working in the field of sexual assault and domestic violence with a mission to end the pain people experience in this deplorable domain. Their unwavering commitment, tenacity, and hard work have heightened awareness, changed attitudes, and created individual successes, yet the goal of eradicating sexual violence remains stubbornly out of reach.

Making Out Like a Virgin: Sex, Desire & Intimacy After Sexual Trauma offers stories in which people have started to own their bodies, to resuscitate and reclaim their lives, to expand possibilities, and to shed secrecy and shame. These stories of personal evolution show the power of vulnerable openness. They affirm the transformation inherent in telling one's truth. They offer models of radical recovery.

There are no mainstream words in the English language for those who have experienced this kind of trauma other than "victim" and "survivor." We desperately need that to change. We need new words to describe people who have reclaimed a life that is flourishing. We need narratives that transcend trauma and imagine a new future. We know there is hope; we know there is *more*. *With Making Out Like a Virgin,* we hope to build momentum for a positive shift.

We envisioned a book that would be a beacon for those who feel they are living without power and are "just making it." Our call for contributions asked for essays that showed life as perfectly imperfect, which would affirm how feelings of doubt, fear, low self-esteem, and being an "imposter" can be acknowledged and then let go. We sought narratives that detail how people built strength and have recovered their capacity for joy. That is exactly what we got. They illuminate that when love prevails, relationships open new worlds.

We were encouraged by the enthusiastic response we received when we vetted the book concept with professionals in the fields of sexuality, sexual assault, and sexual and domestic violence. We were even more thrilled by the conversations we had with potential contributors, each person expressing a deep desire to share their experience moving from victim to survivor and beyond—now thriving in a life they once thought they could never live. We found people who were ready to write these stories and were in turn eager to read about the journey others have taken. Each one wished they had a book like this when they were in the throes of recovery. Positive anticipation grew as the drafts came in and we knew this was a needed addition to the resources currently available.

The 17 contributors in this collection hail from different parts of the world and walks of life. They offer narratives influenced by their differences. While each one has a different perspective, they reveal remarkably similar themes. You may be as surprised as we were to discover that, taken together, their varied paths lead us in the same positive direction. None of them offer up the usual magazine headlines or clickbait listicles for "ten secrets" or "best tips" or "quick results" because there aren't any. But there are common threads that unite them as people who have retrieved feelings of lustful sex, desire, and intimacy and have embraced these feelings.

As you read, there are a few things we ask you to consider. While the writers may have previously written about the violence that happened to them—privately, publicly, or even in a court of law—the retelling of those events is not the focus of their narratives. Any information about their personal experience is shared as context for the changes they made in their lives; some frame the abuse in a broad statement of fact, others weave specifics as needed for the story they tell here. They may not even refer to the whole—or half—of the abuse they have suffered. They may not reveal their name, race, sexual orientation, ethnicity, or other important elements of their idendity. Trauma is one aspect of their lives, not their life story.

These voices represent a snapshot in time, an exploration of the past and present and potential. We hope that they help others to close some doors and to open others. These intimate chronicles offer collective hope for the future for all survivors.

Catriona McHardy,
Cathy Plourde
Editors

FOLDING IN

KEVIN GALLAGHER

Sexual abuse is like a natural disaster. Take for example the catastrophe of flooding: topography and landscape are altered permanently. Heavy rain causes landslides, destroys homes, and swells rivers—even changing their direction. We attempt to defend ourselves from the potential of flooding, or abuse, and yet shit happens. Flooding and abuse are both a part of the human condition.

My own abuse started at around six years old. That's a guess really. I don't remember being terribly aware of calendars, clocks, and seminal moments when I was a young pup. One of my uncles who visited us regularly would come to my room when I was sleeping. This went on for over ten years and was punctuated with other experiences, including abuse by a priest when I was an altar boy and a random sexual assault by two guys when I was 15. Suffice to say that I did not come into my own sexuality by my own choice, or in my own timeframe. It's curious and sad to say that I didn't feel like my body belonged to me. I was a vessel for others' sexual experiences. I was there, present in the rooms, as a bystander and not as a participant.

I was relieved to go to college, to move out of state and have a fresh start. I was known as the "asexual wonder." People came up to me to say, "Are you that Kevin guy who has *never* had sex with anyone—guy or girl? And that you don't even *want* to?" It was a strange badge of honor, and I think I was using this time in my life to reboot: press the Control+Alt+Delete buttons, turn sexuality off, and then hope that when I turned it back on, whatever bug/virus/malware would be gone.

Not a chance. I guess children aren't the only ones who believe in fairytales and magic. I say that I did not have sex with anyone until my junior year of college because this was the first sex that was for *me*. It was sex with someone I wanted to be with, on my time-line, by my choice, as an equal in the transaction. That year I had gone to study abroad in England and my "girlfriend" went to Paris to do the same. Yes, girlfriend. Read between the lines: she was a *girl* who was a *friend*. We did not have a sexual relationship; it was more like affection, like junior high school love, but it passed for a relationship. I traveled to Ireland for Easter weekend and in a pub outside Galway, I met a carpenter 30 years old to my 20. He was cute and funny and bright, my trifecta. We talked and laughed, and he asked me back to his place. I liked him and I was scared shitless. He sensed my anxiety and said that we did not have to do anything, just talk. I could stay if I wanted, on the couch or in his bed. We could touch or we could not. He ended up giving me a backrub and he did not cross any boundaries—a must for me at this point, and also a good sign of his character. By morning we had had sex, and it was good and I was OK. Phew. What a relief.

After Easter, my girlfriend and I met up in Paris. I remember the day vividly. It was cloudy and damp. We sat talking in a booth in a diner that had a jukebox and Debbie Harry, lead singer for Blondie, was singing "The Tide is High." She told me she met a couple and traveled to Greece with them. She ended up being sexual with the wife and had liked it. I felt relief because now I could tell her that I hooked up with a guy in Ireland and I had really liked that. My girlfriend and I were free to love each other and to pursue other love, deeper love, than our own naïve clinging.

So end of story, right? Guy has a positive sexual experience, figures out he's gay, and is good to go. Not exactly. There was no sex after Mr. Ireland for several more years. Eventually I began dating guys. Up until that point I had been confused as to whether I was *really* gay or not. I felt real love for women and wanted to believe that I could have a healthy sexual relationship with one. At the same time, I had only been sexual with men, and that was all that I knew. This made dating and self-discovery a very non-linear process. I was a nice guy, for the most part, and I believed that I deserved to have a good relationship one day. However, I was a 23-year-old dating like a 14-year-old; my dating selections in men were terrible, laughable, even painful, but all educational. One by one, I learned more about how to be a self, a whole person in these encounters: How to have a voice; how to say no (and mean it); and how to ask for what I wanted. I've since come to recognize I am affectionately drawn toward women and erotically oriented toward men. And this realization allows me to feel whole in expressing who I am.

This year is my 30th anniversary with my partner. We met at a dinner party. He was 19 and I was 25. I didn't care for him much, but I liked him enough to play tennis and meet for drinks from time to time. Gradually, we evolved into something else. He is not damaged. He had a profoundly normal sexual development. I was both jealous and intimidated. I remember a few occasions when we were having sex and right in the middle of it, I got up, got dressed, and left without a word. Each time he said, "I'll call you later." So patient and kind. I was such a piece of work that he could have easily moved onto someone without so many hang-ups, triggers, and issues. But he didn't. Both Mr. Ireland and my partner are men of character, men who did not have personal damage that they then took out on others as a way to further the natural disaster.

As a clinical mental health counselor for over 26 years, I have heard hundreds of stories like mine: stories of pain and destruction, stories of growth and recovery. I've seen people whose landscape has been permanently altered, and others who have completely rebuilt their lives. I've met with offenders who were suffering the shame and agony of their actions. I've met with victims who are defined by the event(s) and that label. I don't fully understand why I never told anyone about what was being done to me as a child, a classic problem with abuse. I must have been afraid, knowing that what was happening was wrong, but it was more than fear that kept me silent. I think I didn't have words yet. Words to describe sex, abuse, betrayal, terror, dissociation, and anxiety. Who as a child knows how to describe such complex human dynamics? At that time, I could tell you what I wanted for Christmas and what I had eaten at school that day, but what exactly was I going to say about being abused?

The isolation of suffering and the absence of love can have irrevocable effects. No matter how alone and pained I was as a kid, a teen, or an adult, I knew every day that at least someone, or even many people, loved me. Central to my own recovery is the concept of love. I don't call having sex "making love." I think sex and love are very different. By this I mean that love is verb, an action taken toward another, and not necessarily sexual.

To feel loved, valued, and respected is the only path that I can see toward reclaiming intimacy. I'm not talking about romantic or erotic love since that can be fleeting. Love *from* others and *toward* others was an essential element in my feeling whole again as a sexual being. I believe my love toward others is what comes first, and in return I get back tenfold what I give. Maybe this is why I'm a therapist; my job is to care.

I've come up with a "dented can" theory as a way to help me conceptualize my past abuse. Back in the day, there used to be a section of the grocery store that sold cans that were dented from shipping or poor stacking, often missing their labels. You could buy them for a dime or a quarter and take a chance on what you were getting. That's how I feel as a survivor of abuse. I am a dented can, not as pristine and well labeled as the other cans on the shelves. The contents are still intact. The same good food exists inside. I'm not suggesting that I'm damaged goods; rather, I am a container with a unique shape, a changed package with perfectly fine contents. And if you, with sensitivity and tolerance, can appreciate what I have to offer—kindness, dedication, humor, thoughtfulness, commitment, and hard work—I will appreciate these qualities in you.

I had always wondered, "Why me? Why was I abused?" Bad luck? Reincarnation gone afoul? Sins of the father? Well, one day my therapist said,

I have to tell you something. I would not say this if you were not
a therapist yourself, because I'd fear what you would think. When
I saw you in my schedule today, I was excited to see you. I don't
have this kind of reaction to all my clients. And it made me think
that this might help explain why you were abused. You know when
there is a litter of puppies and people come to see them, there is
always one that everyone wants? I think that is you. I think you
were wanted for all the qualities that make you special, and you
were taken advantage of by men who wanted those things in their
own lives and were trying to steal them from you.

In my profession I witness abuse in all its ugliness—people
who have done simply terrible things to others, and people who
have had miserable things done to them. I hear the cries and watch
the tears of people longing to be unburdened by their pain, regret,
sadness, and rage. When people expect me to "fix them," I conjure
up a cooking metaphor for this particular challenge.

Some recipes call for folding in ingredients. I never understood
this concept. How can you *fold* an ingredient in? Doesn't it have to
be thoroughly mixed and become part of the whole? My partner,
the chef in the family, tells me that folding in means that you only
move the ingredients around, you don't blend or beat or fully mix
the contents. Perhaps recovering from abuse is not about letting the
abuse get so integrated that the whole mixture—you—becomes con-
taminated by the abuse. Perhaps I can gently fold my experience in,
knowing that it's a part of me, but it's not something to define me. I
am not *abuse*; I was *abused*.

In our 30 years together, I've found that in order to be the kind of cook—or the kind of survivor of abuse—that I want to be, I have to be gentle, patient, and attentive, like my partner is with me.

We fold together well.

Psychotherapist by day and storyteller by night, Kevin Gallagher attempts to use his solid Irish background for the forces of good. He is a private practitioner in Burlington, Vermont, working primarily with young adults and families, and does storytelling to raise money for community nonprofits. From his perspective, stories provide the connective means through which we grow and change.

BREATHING COMPASSION
LYNNETTE E. HARPER

I look back now and can parse out what was happening, but in the individual moments all I knew is I'd freeze and tell myself: "I can't do this." After being raped at 18, relationships were too scary, too intimate.

I wooed men into bed because in bed I could control everything. That's what I'd done my whole life: Sex was the tool I wielded to seize control, and that control created a cocoon of safety around me. But even with control, I still disassociated. I wasn't there. Emotionally, I was two zip codes away from my physical body.

I fucked inappropriate men: ones who were too old for me, addicts, married men, predators. Men who didn't care about anything except that I was young, blond, and willing. They wanted me, and they didn't care for me, and we had that in common—I didn't care for myself, either.

I never considered that how I was using my body could make me feel even worse than I usually felt. I longed for kindness, love, connection, and I didn't understand that heartless sex was the wrong route to that kind of attention. I just thought I was wrong. If the only thing I and others seemed to value about me—my body—couldn't make me feel better about myself, then everything about me was all wrong, and I was pretty much doomed.

I married a boy I barely knew because he was my way out. By attaching myself to him, I saw a clear avenue to a world of respectability and decency: a shelter, a relationship to be proud of. Yet inside I still carried that lack of care and that lack of me-ness. I finally had culturally appropriate "safety" in being married, yet it didn't give me any idea of what to do next. I'd never been shown or taught anything about intimacy or even told that I had worth.

I met him in San Francisco when I was a nanny and he was in the military. Looking back, he was my surrogate dad. His history even ran parallel with my father's: Each lost a parent at a young age; had an addicted surviving parent; grew up with an unstable childhood; went into the military young; and became addicted to alcohol—although they were nice drunks and people liked them. Nice drunks can get away with a lot.

I deferred to my husband completely, but he was an uneducated alcoholic who had no desire to run the show. He wanted me to just do everything—and I did. I did all the things a good Christian wife should do: Dropped out of a secular university; stopped working to make dinner every night and keep house; went to weekly and sometimes thrice-weekly Bible study; attended every church function; went to a women's Bible retreat; tithed; volunteered; smiled; wore modest clothing. All to prove to my husband that I was worthy of his attention.

The only problem was that I was angry. Very, very angry, every single day.

Few people knew this, though. I was cheerful and kind. I took cupcakes to neighbors, watched friend's babies so they could have date nights, and gave rides to hitchhikers. I carried myself with such confidence that people kept mistaking me for a person with authority. Students at the Bible college thought I was an instructor. People at church thought I was a pastor's wife. Once, at a women's church retreat, I was pulled into the leadership council and it took the pastor's wife to convince the other women I wasn't a church leader. I exuded competence, although I was also terrified to be exposed as a fraud. What ran like a river underneath my capable façade was simmering rage.

Anger was the way I kept people around me subdued and in line. Anger was my jetpack. It thrust me out of the infinitesimally small hometown in which I finished high school. It hurled me free of the wreckage of my family, a rape, an unwanted pregnancy, and an abortion. It slung me into opportunity after opportunity. Anger and rage catapulted me forward even as I was angry and rage-filled at myself for doing things that made me feel so stupid.

My mom had shown me clearly that you stay in your marriage. No matter how bad it gets, you stay. If you stay, you win, because no one can talk about you. You're the good girl. No one wants a bad girl. Bad girls are dirty. They're whores. They're women who steal other people's men.

I spent twelve years of married life living out my childhood, living out my parents' lives, living out the entire belief system that I wasn't worth love, I had no right to ask for it, I had to earn it, and I probably would never be able to. It was my responsibility to make things work. Mine. If things were shit it was because I was not trying hard enough. It was my fault, my problem, and failure was my true self.

At a certain point, my anger wasn't enough to save me. I was a bad girl. I didn't know how to be anything else.

I left my marriage on 9/11. The entire world was trying to get back home. I was trying to never go home again.

∴

June 10, 2015, meditation retreat

My left thigh is on fire. I am kneeling with my feet tucked perfectly under my butt, hands resting on my thighs, palms up, eyes closed, breathing with the counting man whose quiet voice barely rises above the sound of traffic from one story below.

I follow the breath counts dutifully, while the voices in my head maraud around pointing out everything that's pissing me off in the moment: Why are these meditation cushions only as thick as a piece of paper? Who picked out this music—was there truly nothing more annoying on the market? Doesn't iTunes have a recording of a roll of nickels banging around in a dryer? Because that would be preferable to whatever is playing right now. How much longer is this going to last? This is awful. I can't believe I am paying to learn how to hyperventilate. I was doing this in eighth grade in Todd McVicker's garage. We'd bend over and pant, then stand up quickly, in hopes of fainting. I did not have to come to a foreign country to learn this.

On the third day of class I said during check-in, "I'm not sure I'm healthy enough to be doing this. I think I should go get my shit together and come back in a few months."

The teacher laughed a full-on laugh with her head thrown back and then looked me dead in the eye and said, not unkindly, "You are right where you are supposed to be."

Having spent many years on therapists' couches clutching tissues and crying, I thought I was pretty solid. I was a licensed massage therapist, I had taken yoga training in Thailand, and I was an old hand in meditation classes. My body and I weren't exactly best friends, but we could at least recognize each other on the street. I liked sex, eating, drinking, hiking, and other bodily pleasures. I was fine. And my mind and I are one and the same, aren't we? No problem there. But then there were the other voices.

I always knew I had voices in my head and it wasn't until this class that I realized what assholes they were. Absolute terrors! They knew my weak spots and went after them with fervor. I say "voices" but it was mostly just one voice, you know the one that sounds weirdly like one or both of your parents when they're unusually disappointed in you? That one. The same internal voice that reminds you that every mistake is the one that proves you, I mean me, *me*, I am incompetent beyond reason, that every bad dating decision is proof I will be bitter and die alone, leaving my corpse for the cats, which I don't even have, to gnaw on.

This voice spurred me on in life while never offering safety, only judgment. I can always recognize this voice; it's lacking in any compassion or kindness. It is hard and sharp and quick. It is usually the first to speak up. Under ordinary circumstances I can distract myself or ignore it, but not while meditating.

Sitting and listening in on your thoughts isn't as easy as it sounds. This voice is so terribly unkind it's uncomfortable to sit with. I don't want to admit this voice is mine. It belittles and judges and makes sure I always "know my place." The practice of sitting meditation helped me realize that this voice had been on in an endless loop in my head for years. Something as simple as trying to bring in too many bags of groceries at once and dropping one bag would be met with an internal, "Jesus! You are such an idiot!" It never occurred to me that was abusive. I just thought it was normal—if I didn't keep myself on track, who would?

When I first began to notice my thoughts and heard their disdain, I asked myself, "Would you say that to a three-year-old?" Merely imagining it would make my gut drop. I'd say things to myself that would be outright violence if you said them to a child. But I had no problem saying or thinking these things about myself.

That small question shifted my awareness and helped me find kinder ways to relate to myself, and by default to others. No longer do I engage in that typical banter with other women about wishing I could lose weight, or what to do about my wrinkles. A dear co-worker said to me the other day that she was getting lines around her mouth and eyes and was considering fillers. My honest reply was, "I have always loved how much expression you show when you talk and seeing you laugh is one of my favorite things, especially when it's a hard day at work."

Being with my thoughts in a non-judgmental way has encouraged me to engage with other people honestly and kindly—including myself. Being aware of my own mind has helped me so much on my journey to self-compassion. And self-compassion has loosened the parts of me that were always on guard, not letting me feel the world very deeply.

It turns out that each tiny pivot toward my true self brings me closer to my sensuality. Every moment I can be open and kind and honest brings me deeper into what I need to feel secure in relationships. Every breath brings me home to my body, and it's a home that's safe for me to inhabit. My life is so much richer, and my senses so much more alert, the more aware I become. Something as simple as a slice of apricot tastes complex and vivid. I notice the texture of a sleeping lover's hair against the skin of my arm. I'm awake in such a new way, and I feel lucky, and grateful.

Sometimes, I still have extraordinarily harsh thoughts. I caught myself in the reflection of a window the other day and my immediate reaction was, "You have the flattest ass of any woman on earth." Seriously, it was in my head before I passed my reflection, but I was aware of it and instead of letting it just go by unheeded, I was able to take a deep breath and say quietly, "That was one fast put-down, and I do not accept that I have the flattest ass on earth!"

Meditation brings awareness to what I think about myself. That awareness slowly helps me heal in quiet internal ways and I am learning how to heal. It is such a profound journey and I do not think there is an end to it. Every single breath is an opportunity to come home: a home where I truly care for myself, where I show myself compassion, where I experience pleasure, and where I heal.

I still hate sitting on my knees. I still have mean thoughts about the annoying music, yet each week I go to meditation and I breathe, and I learn to be gentler with my thoughts. Each week, I ask if there is different music we can listen to and each week they tell me no. I still kneel down, take that first deep breath, and fall quietly in love with myself. I have found my way home to my sensuality through breath, gorgeous flat ass and all.

Lynnette E. Harper is a librarian living in Dubai who diabolically loves pit bulls. She has been a cosmetologist, licensed massage therapist, ESL teacher, yoga instructor, heavy equipment operator, and children's librarian. She worked in an industrial plumbing warehouse and managed crews working in materials at the South Pole. She has never been published and has no idea what she is doing with her life, but she enjoys it all the same.

Freedom At My Fingertips

Sarah Mell

In the summer of 1996, I spent my days waiting tables and my nights, late nights, late-late nights, and early mornings hanging out with Kate. Single mom with a horrible ex, an adorable two-year-old daughter, small apartment, charming smile, silly sense of humor, nurturing touch… Kate…

Kate was the first person I came out to who actually heard me and said it was OK; Kate was also the first person who told me "it" wasn't my fault. Before Kate, I had kept my mouth shut about what Grandpa did. I had kept my mouth shut since I was six and my parents decided that "it" didn't happen. *Don't talk about "it." Pretend "it" wasn't real. Keep everything "normal."* I didn't know what normal was. Kate saw me, loved me, and it was good. Kate felt normal.

We weren't together, so to speak; Kate wasn't a lesbian and didn't want to date me, but I knew that she loved me. Kate was the first woman I slept with—the first female body I touched in ways I had never touched myself. I never, ever touched myself. While other kids worried about getting caught "she-bopping," I was horrified at the thought of touching myself "down there." That was not a space for me, but for others. It always had been. A space for my Grandfather. A space to show neighborhood boys. A space to let the middle school boys explore while I stared at the sky. A space that was meant to please everyone else but me.

That summer propelled me into therapy and a nose piercing — rites of passage in a young queer survivor's life — and I returned to college that fall having discovered sex with a woman. Silence was my enemy and hiding didn't fit. But I hadn't discovered how all of this was alive in the sinews of my own body. I remained a stranger to my needs and pleasure. Then, I found Sophia...

Sophia sat across the table at the Steak n' Shake as I sipped my hot chocolate. I blushed at her knowing gaze and knew I was in for it. We spent the next two years navigating the ins and outs of a closeted love affair, praying to Jesus to forgive us our sins and convincing our friends and family that our friendship flourished because of our mutual love for music and literature. The make-believe bedroom in our two-bedroom apartment was full of furniture that slumbered without us, covered in the hair of our cat, Byron.

I enjoyed sex with Sophia, reveled in orgasm for the first time in my young life, practiced comfort and warmth, passion and exhaustion, thrill and silliness. We were each other's first everything, or at least mostly everything. Through the vehicle of her tender and safe caress, Sophia helped me see that my body was a place where I, too, could find pleasure. Always, still, to be kept secret; always, still, full of shame. *Don't let the neighbors know. Don't let our parents find out. Deny our curious friends. Pray for a way to love one another that doesn't equal sin.*

After a couple of years, the silence about our secret life took its toll. Just one county north of where we lived, people were fired from their jobs for coming out. We couldn't risk the exposure of being us. I was 22 and exhausted from the fight. Exhausted from once again being asked to pretend "it" wasn't happening, "it" didn't exist: it, us, love. I crumbled and the relationship followed suit.

I was alone after two years, two months, and eleven days of a love that had transformed me, and yet I was unable to break through the shame. That's what a closet will do. That's what stolen childhoods like mine will do. But I'm not here to dwell on what happened when I was four, when I was five, when I was six; I'm not here to detail how those moments in the basement with Grandpa permeated my first relationship, or explain why guilt, disgrace, and a love of Jesus leaked from our eyes while Sophia and I held hands in the dark movie theater—the one place we could love each other in public. I'm here to talk about the lessons I learned after that. I'm here to talk about Renee...

What's a newly single lesbian in Kalamazoo, Michigan to do with herself but stumble into the town's one gay bar to try and dance it out? That's what I was doing the night I met Renee. Lenny Kravitz blasting through the speakers; me in my SPAM t-shirt, over-alls, and blue Chucks; Renee dancing, lithe and free....

"Hey."

"Hey."

"I like the way you dance."

"Thanks."

"Wanna dance with me?"

"Yeah, I think I'd like that."

I remember thinking that she looked like a fairy. Like Peter Pan had finally come to rescue me, and had sent Tinker Bell ahead to make sure I was ready for my escape to Neverland. I remember the freckles on her nose as she danced close to me, our faces and our mouths nearly meeting, then turning away just before touching.

"Renee." —*pointing to herself.*

"Sarah." —*pointing to myself.*

"I don't think I've seen you here before."

"I haven't been in a couple of years."

"Single?"

"I am now."

"Recent?"

"Does it matter?"

"No."

"The song's over, wanna get some air?"

"Sure."

The back deck at the Zoo was always my favorite part of that bar. We sipped cool, tall glasses of water under swaying maples full of twinkle lights, the bass of the next song vibrating the boards beneath our feet—or maybe I was shaking from the nerves. What did we talk about? School? Where we grew up? Did we talk at all? I can't recall now, but I remember smiling and Renee placing the dampness of her water glass against my cheek when I flushed from a compliment she gave. I was being wooed and flattered and I didn't know what to do with this person who was full of joy and freedom. It excited me to think I could get that close to letting go. She was a mirror image, distorted by a hippie sensibility and a freedom to love herself, and seeing the possibilities of me without the shame, without the hurt, without anything but joy. Renee and her freckled nose. Renee and her pixie hair a slightly darker shade of dirty blonde than my own. Renee and her petite, scrappy frame. Renee and her armpit hair, her delicate chin, her spritely spirit, her patchouli and pot aroma.

I can't remember if I took her back to my place that night, or if I stayed with her in the four-bedroom Victorian she shared with three roommates. I can't remember if we slept together, or if we maybe went our separate ways for a good night's sleep. I can't remember when I decided that she would be my summer plans. We spent hours driving around Kalamazoo County; getting lost and wandering through graveyards; and sitting on her front porch while I played my guitar, Savannah (she's the one who named it), and she smoked a bowl and philosophized about love. We weren't in love. We knew that. And we thought that was lovely.

Renee freaked out my conservative Christian roommates. She didn't wear deodorant on her unshaven underarms and she talked about socialism like it was a good idea. My roommates were fascinated and concerned about me. I was fascinated, too. Renee loved life and let everyone around her know it. And, she was unabashedly sexual in ways that had never occurred to me.

When I held Renee I realized what it must be like to hold me. We were standing in her bedroom and there was a party happening on the other side of the door. I pulled her five-foot-five, agile and delicate, strong and sensual frame against my own and thought, "This is what I feel like. This is what my body feels like in another woman's arms!" I was thrilled and terrified. She was teaching me to love *me*.

That night, after hours of playing, laughing, crying out, and transforming our bodies into positions and shapes that I had never dreamed of, we finally lay still in the balance of her tiny twin mattress telling stories. She told me of her journeys to China and the man she loved there; about a childhood in Minnesota and a family that mostly understood her, but couldn't wrap their heads around her need for travel and exploration. I told her about Kate, Sophia, and my family back in Michigan, about the sweeping beauty of my childhood by the lake and the crushing shame of my Grandfather's hands. We talked a lot about hands that night. Hands that can heal and hands that can hurt. Our fingers intertwined and drew circles on each other's palms, bellies, thighs, and then Renee guided our hands, my hand, toward the one part of my body that was off limits to me.

"What's wrong?"

"I can't."

"It's because of when you were a kid. It's OK."

(She slowly moves our hands lower.)

"Stop. Please."

"OK, OK. It's OK."

(I am crying and she is holding me.)

"I will never make you do anything you don't want to do."

"Thank you."

As Renee dropped off to sleep, her nose nuzzled into my neck and her breathing deep and steady, I lay awake staring at the nails in her ceiling. *Why had I stopped her? What's the big deal? It's my own body! My body!* I was frustrated, angry, scared, and exhausted. It felt as though I was on the precipice of a monumental shift, if I could only take that first step.

For the next several weeks, I took baby steps toward releasing the shame that kept me separated from my body. Little things. Taking more care to notice in the shower or when using the bathroom. Resting my hand there, over my PJs, as I fell asleep at night. Asking questions of Renee about it after lovemaking. I wanted to know more; I wanted Renee to teach me.

Saturday morning, front porch, coffee and cigarettes — mine tobacco, hers not; conversation:

"Renee, when was the first time you masturbated?"

"Oh wow, I don't know…maybe when I was ten or so."

"Ten years old!"

"I think that's pretty normal."

"Wow."

"It was normal for me. It's OK that it wasn't for you. You'll get there; I have faith."

Tuesday evening, car ride, me driving, Renee with her leg out the passenger window; conversation:

"I can feel the breeze on my bits!"

"Is that a good thing?"

"Absolutely! You should try it!"

"Maybe not while I'm driving."

"Then let me drive."

Thursday afternoon, random ice cream shop, middle of Nowheresville, Michigan; conversation:

"But what would I do?"

"What you do with me."

"But I don't think I could. I mean, logistically."

"You'll figure it out. You do what feels good and let your mind drift off a bit. Don't think about it so much, just go with the flow."

"Go with the flow…yeah…you're high."

She probably was high, but she was probably right and I wanted so badly to believe her. So, the following Wednesday, after an eight-hour shift at the greenhouse, two cigarettes and a beer in the backyard, a long hot shower, and a big self-pep-talk...I was goin' in. No one else home, no plans, no distractions, just me and my... well, me.

I remember lying very still under a single sheet, my back hot and damp from my shower and the humidity of the summer evening.

I remember closing my eyes because when I kept them open I stared at the overhead light that was covered with dust and couldn't stop thinking about it needing to be cleaned.

I remember trying to focus my brain on someone "sexy"— Renee at first, then Sophia, then all the way back to Kate, and on to any number of people I found attractive.

I remember finally just letting my mind wander at the same pace as my wandering hand; my fingers cool against my belly.

I remember smiling. Lots of smiling. And then... joy. Joy and freedom and smiling. Images flashed through my mind's eye—the lake, Sophia's dimpled cheek, Renee the night we met— joy and freedom and smiling—I did it! I was so present, so myself, so proud. I immediately rolled over, grabbed my phone, and called Renee.

"Hello?"

"I did it!"

"Hello? Who is this?"

"It's me, Sarah. I did it! *I masturbated!"*

"What? Oh my god! I'm so proud of you! How was it?"

"It was amazing! You were so right! Thank you thank you thank you thank you!"

"No need to thank me, I'm just so happy for you! You're beautiful and that's wonderful!"

"Sorry to bother you with a random phone call—I just wanted you to know."

"Thank you for telling me. I have people over right now, but I'll see you soon, OK?"

"Yes, of course, thank you, soon, I'll see you soon! Bye!"

"Bye."

I rolled back over in my queen-sized bed and made sheet angels with my arms and legs, beaming like a child in her first snowstorm. This was an entirely new world. A world of my own making. I felt so free, and sleepy, and I promptly drifted off as the evening's remaining sunlight streamed through my window.

I was proud of my accomplishment and unabashedly told my roommates, my coworkers, and complete strangers. OK, maybe not strangers, but I felt everyone should know, in case they didn't already, that *masturbation was grand*. When I next saw Renee, we celebrated by having sex, loudly, with lots of laughter and acrobatics. She asked if I wanted to show her—no, that was one step too far for my newfound freedom. It would take years before I masturbated in front of another person. (That's its own magical experience, for another time, another story.)

It was an early August afternoon when I swung by Renee's to pick her up for one of our last adventures. Summer was drawing to a close and soon I would be moving to Vermont. Her roommate answered the door, the aroma of pot heavy on her clothes and in the air:

"Hey, I'm here to pick up Renee."

"Ummm… she's not here."

"Oh, OK. Well, I guess she forgot."

"No, I mean…she's, like, gone."

"What do you mean, gone?"

"Like, she doesn't live here anymore."

"Wait, what? Where did she go?"

"Ummm…"

"Do you know how to reach her?"

"Nope."

"Oh. OK. Well. Thanks."

"Yup."

I slowly descended the porch steps. She was gone. Just like that. No goodbye. No contact info. Nothing. It was so "Renee" of her; always the free spirit, there was no pinning her down. As I drove home, swinging by the liquor store to pick up packing boxes for my impending move, I briefly wondered if she had been real, this pixie with the freckles on her nose and freedom in her fingertips. I grinned, thinking of how such a short and frivolous romance had completely transformed me.

I was about to launch on the biggest adventure of my 23 years: moving across the country to a state that was talking about letting gay folks marry—unheard of in my neck of the conservative Midwest woods—where I was finally going to be able to be fully me— out, open, no secrets, no denials, no limits. Renee was my compass as I embarked on that 1000-mile crossing to the next stage of me. The lessons she taught me in how to touch myself, to revel in the beauty I hadn't seen before and to call it my own, put me on a path to sexual experiences I otherwise couldn't have imagined.

It's been 16 years since the summer I learned to masturbate. Partners have come and gone. I have had sex that was earth-shattering and sex that was just meant to help us fall asleep; sex that made me cry from the intensity of the connection and sex that had me giggling when physics got in the way of our best laid plans; sex that tried to save an engagement and sex that celebrated a marriage.

I like to think these moments have been possible because of that late-June evening back in Kalamazoo when I met Renee and started a two-month fling that ended with me recognizing that shame and sex aren't synonymous, and that freedom should always be a part of the equation—freedom to choose who gets to go on this ride with me; freedom to express my desires openly and passionately; freedom to talk about what I want and to fulfill those wants with or without a partner; freedom to explore fantasies and whims; and freedom to find joy in all of it.

Sarah Mell is an educator, performer, and activist who has spent the last decade helping people of all ages, backgrounds, and genders talk about sex. She is forever indebted to the mentoring and training she received as a sexuality educator at Planned Parenthood of Northern New England; it helped to craft the confident survivor identity that is so integral to her living life out loud. She can be found on stage, in the classroom, and often dancing in the kitchen of her home in Vermont with her inspirational wife and four-legged family.

PERFECT KISS

TERI WEST

It's my 14th birthday and the last day of 8th grade. Mr. S has offered me a ride home in his sporty convertible. On the way there, he says he needs to make a quick stop at an apartment where he is doing some carpentry work. We get into a private elevator for the penthouse apartment but halfway up, Mr. S pulls the emergency stop button. He looks directly at me, and says, "I haven't given you a birthday kiss yet. Can I do that?"

"Okay," I reply, confused, thinking he will give me a peck on the cheek.

My heart is pounding and an endless loop of "Oh my god" is stuck in my head. I am there, but I am outside of myself looking at my disembodied self kissing Mr. S, my junior high school science teacher. My science teacher, who is having an affair with my mother; my science teacher, who is married with two children. My fingers tingle. The flapping birds in my stomach move to my heart

and are in ecstatic flight. I watch myself from the outside and then
my senses are magnified on my mouth: his lips, soft and gentle;
his tongue, wet and smooth. I am detached from time and space as
his tongue snakes its way through my mouth, across my teeth, and
under my tongue, forever imprinting his smell, his taste, and the
feel of that kiss on my soul. That kiss becomes the kiss by which all
other kisses will be judged. I stop breathing and lose my bearings;
I am caught between an encroachment and a gift, repulsion and
attraction, presence and absence, in the moment and miles from it.

On my tiptoes, I put my arms around his shoulders to steady
myself. I finally take a breath, and then I step back, dizzy and alive.

∴

My husband steps out of the bathroom with his face clean-
shaven. My heart shifts into high gear; I clench my jaw and turn my
fists into balls. Why am I feeling so anxious? Why do I feel a sudden
panic when I look at his shaven face? His deep set, dark eyes now
pop from his face against his newly creamy-white cheek; the cleft
on his chin seems to mock me; and the curl of his top lip, no longer
hidden behind his mustache, smiles at me. I have never known him
without a beard, and his face at this moment becomes the face of the
man who seduced me many times over the course of a year when I
was a child. I take a deep breath, nod my head to the uncomfortable
feeling I am having, slap a coy smile on my face, and deliberately
put that memory in the corner of my mind. I cup his face in my
hands and stroke his chin. We are cheek to cheek as I gently caress
my lips across his face and land them in a passionate kiss.

I don't tell him that his face reminds me of Mr. S. I don't tell him for several months, in fact, because I am embarrassed, ashamed of my feelings, and worried about what he might think. What could he possibly think after 15 years of marriage? That there is something wrong with me because I still think of Mr. S after 38 years, that the image and memory of Mr. S has invaded my mind, and reproduces like kudzu? Is it that insidious? Am I being overly dramatic? Have I subconsciously (or consciously) married a man who looks like the man who seduced me when I was in junior high school? Why is this still, *still* coming back to me? This feeling gives me pause: I came to terms with my sexual trauma, didn't I? But here it is again, in the guise of a clean shave, rearing its face at me, and demanding that I confront it. Oh you demons of the past! Be gone! *Please?*

The sense that my husband reminds me of Mr. S has lurked in the shadows of my mind since I met him. Same dark hair and deep brown eyes, hairy body, and pudgy well-manicured fingers. He has a stereotypical Jewish boy look about him, and a similar — what's that space between the nose and the upper lip? Yeah, that, whatever that's called. Plus, they are both adept at science, have birthdays in early July, and went to college in Connecticut. If those things mean anything. The similarities end there, but Mr. S has never left my subconscious. The many sexual encounters I had with him over the course of that one formative year of my life are recalled in every sexual experience I have had since — he is stuck there forever as my personal creation myth for what men and sex are. It is not news to me that Mr. S has had a lasting, formative influence on the development of my sexual expression and pleasure. This realization has taken me decades to recognize, to understand, to accept, and to control. And the repercussions continue to reverberate through my life in unexpected and unanticipated ways.

The through-line of my adult sexual fantasy life has always been about being submissive: the vulnerable, weak, shy girl who is taken by the powerful man; the voluptuous, naive 17-year-old at the doctor's office; the sacrificial, pubescent child who is gang raped over a flat rock by the tribal men to please the gods. My adolescent fantasies about Mr. S were relatively tame; I thought about him holding me down, or touching me while I lay quiet and still. One late night when he was with my mother, I left the hall light shining through my open door onto my bed. I hiked up my nightgown to my ass and kicked the covers to my ankles. I was wearing underpants, but I wanted him to see my body when he stepped out of my mother's room. I waited up, pretending to be asleep when he stepped out of her room. I heard him pause at my door. He didn't come in that time. There were other times when he did. The issue that I struggled with for so many years was whether I had brought that violation on myself through my masturbation fantasies. That was the source of my guilt and shame: I had made my fantasy become a reality in that magical way that children will things into being.

I never gave voice to my fantasies with my partners; I thought they were deviant. I was ashamed of them, and ashamed of myself for having them because they were tightly linked to my sexual trauma. But I needed to think of these fantasies to have an orgasm. I was having sex without communicating my desires, without sharing my fantasies, and without telling my partner what I liked and didn't like.

Being silent was not the only thing that kept me from having a healthy and positive sex life. I had also lied to my mother for ten years about what her boyfriend had done to me. Telling her the truth, more than a decade later, was complicated because she had "discovered" it while it was happening.

I was visiting cousins for a few days at the end of July, the summer between junior high and high school. One afternoon while swimming in their pool, the phone rang. My aunt called me from the kitchen and told me there was a call for me from my friend, Michael. I was confused: Michael and I were friends from elementary school, but we drifted into different groups in junior high. Why would he be calling? How did he even know where I was? With a towel draped across my shoulders and chest, I held the receiver to my ear, "Michael?"

The voice on the other end did not belong to Michael. "This is Mr. S. Are you alone?" I took the call in the den and called out to my aunt to hang up the extension in the kitchen. Mr. S continued, "I want you to just listen right now. Don't say anything, and don't panic. Your mother found a diary where you wrote things about you and me. I want you to answer just 'yes' or 'no' because I know you can't talk." He paused and then asked, "Do you want to tell your mother the truth?"

My heart was pounding; I couldn't breathe, and my hands began to tremble. I most certainly did not want to tell my mother. He asked if I knew what I would say to her. What? What? What? My mind went blank and a white cloud surrounded my field of vision. I felt like I was going to faint and needed to pull myself together. *My mother had read my diary about the things I had done with*

*Mr. S: kissing; going for rides with him in his car; touching me in the most
private of places; smoking pot.* I was fucked.

"You don't need to panic," he said. "I have an idea. Tell your
mother that you have a crush on me and what you wrote in your
diary is just a fantasy — that you are writing a fantasy story."

That was a lie, of course. What else did I have? How could I
get out of this? When I got home my mother confronted me. I gave
her my story. I looked her square in her green eyes, my chin slightly
lowered, and promised her that "nothing happened." I swore to
God in the way that a 14-year-old girl does when she's caught in
a lie — eyes squinting hard, pressing all the emphasis on the word
swear, and squeezing the lie through the tightly pressed corners of
my mouth so as no truth could escape. Looking back on it now —
as the mother of adolescents — my lie was obvious. But the mind
believes what it wants to believe.

After days of interrogation, picking apart my journal entries,
being grounded, calling me a bitch, and slapping me in the face, my
mother gave up her fight and tossed my diary on my bed. "You can
have this back," she said with an air of disgust and resignation. She
continued her affair with Mr. S; I tore up the incriminating pages of
my book, flushing the evidence through the stinking sewer system
of New York City. I ripped and tore and stifled my cries of rage,
loneliness, and misery. I would never, EVER, tell my mother or
anyone else the truth. I would never write about it or tell about it
and no one would ever find out what a terrible person I was. I shut
myself up in a shell for years.

*April 1978. I'm doing something wrong. I'm a bad person. I'm
deviant and rotten. There is something wrong with me. I'm not*

smart. I'm not beautiful. But he likes me! And he wants me! It feels so good, and I want to feel good, but it is wrong. No one will accept me. No one will understand how good it feels to like me in THAT way. And if I don't go with him then he won't like me. And if I tell anyone they will make it stop. I don't want it to stop.

It took me a long time to accept the fact that I had wanted the pleasure Mr. S had given me. Even as I write it now I am still appalled at my own declaration of this fact. Why is it so hard to admit this publicly? I have admitted it to myself for decades. I have talked about it in hundreds of hours of therapy sessions. I have told my closest confidantes as well as my newest acquaintances. And yet, it still felt like my dirty little secret: I liked what he did. I wanted him! (There, I said it.) He gave me orgasms and made me feel so good. (There, I said it even harder!) He made me feel visible and desired at a time in my life when I felt invisible and unwanted. I wanted him to want me, to kiss me, to love me. I gave him my body in exchange for his love. And, of course, I thought he loved me back. That was a powerful feeling. The pleasure won out over all the bad feelings. I couldn't stop it; I didn't want it to stop. And yet I felt deep shame and guilt about it. Shame because he was my science teacher and I knew that was wrong, and guilt because I was having a secret affair with my mother's boyfriend.

When I understood my motivations, my immaturity and powerlessness, and the circumstances of my life, I let go of the guilt. Letting go of the shame has been a much more difficult process.

September 1983. If my friends know they will shun me. If my mother knows, she will banish me from her life and see it as a betrayal. If I stay silent and keep the secret, I am betraying myself and will be miserable and unhappy for the rest of my life.

My final encounter with Mr. S occurred about two weeks after my mother read my diary, in the summer of 1978, after I graduated from junior high when I was 15 years old. I told my mother I was going to spend the afternoon at the pool and instead met Mr. S for a secret visit to his parents' apartment. He laid a towel down on their king size bed and undressed me, asking if I had started getting my period yet. I had not, and would not reach menarche until three years later when I was almost 17. He took off his pants, unbuttoned his shirt, lay down on the bed, lifted me on top of him, and carefully and painfully fucked me. When he was done, he handed me the towel and my clothes and directed me to go into the bathroom and clean up the blood that was smeared across my thighs. I looked at my swollen and blotchy face in the mirror, splashed water on it, and swallowed my tears. I walked home with my insides burning and toilet tissue stuffed into my panties to absorb the blood. My teeth chattered in the 90-degree summer heat and I hurt so much I could barely walk. That was my first fuck, and my last visit with Mr. S. I stopped seeing him after that. Or maybe he stopped seeing me.

After six years of being lonely and depressed, I told a high school friend about what happened. I swore her to secrecy, still fearful that people would think I was a terrible person. I had fooled everyone except myself into believing I was a good girl; I wasn't ready to change that. My friend pulled me into a big hug and cursed Mr. S saying, "What a fucking prick he is! You ought to cut off his penis!" I laughed and then cried.

Although my friend reassured me that it wasn't my fault, those words echoed hollow in my ears for several more years as I told other friends. My friends didn't know my heart; they didn't know the deep desire I had for Mr. S. Nonetheless, I feasted on the sympathy and expressions of love from friends who marveled at how strong I was and how much I had endured. I never imagined that something I felt so awful about could elicit such love and support, yet I still felt unworthy of love and doubted that I would find lasting happiness in a committed relationship because of what I had done. It took many years and hours in therapy, reflecting on and analyzing my life and primary relationships before the words "it wasn't your fault" started to feel real. I had defined myself and my relationships through sexual trauma and the lies I told to cover it up. Telling my true story has been a process of redefining myself—putting it out there, naming it, taking control of it, and hearing how the people who I love react and respond. But the person I most needed to tell was my mother.

Fast forward from that last year of junior high: I was two years out of college, ten years after the trauma, and I had the means to see a therapist. Two years of therapy helped me understand and make sense of my childhood, of why and how I became entangled with Mr. S. It brought me much closer to forgiving myself and coming clean with my mother.

May 1987. The big event of the weekend was that I told my mother my secret. Told her about Mr. S, the child molester, and she reacted in a way that shocked me. She wasn't angry. I had thought so much that she would be angry. I was so scared to tell her because I didn't know what she would do. But she wasn't angry. She came

*over to comfort me. Maybe she didn't want to show her anger in
front of [my therapist]. I know she was very hurt and angry at
Mr. S and she is stuck now because she doesn't know what to do.
Slowly, slowly, I am starting to feel better now that I have told her.
The worst is over.*

I no longer had to worry that my mother would find out. I *did*
worry about what she would do with the information. She was
stuck because she was in love with Mr. S and he was still in her life.
I hated this man who had violated me and taken advantage of my
vulnerability. I did not understand her lack of action. Instead of
subjugating my feelings to hers, I wrote to her with an ultimatum:
she could have a relationship with Mr. S or she could have a relationship with me. I was worried that she would choose him over
me. I was angry and felt guilty that I was in the position to make her
choose between me and the man she was in love with, even though
he was a duplicitous scumbag. I was not used to exerting my power
and communicating my needs like that, but it was a risk I needed
to take. A week or so after receiving my letter, she told me that the
affair was over.

∴

Although my sexual initiation taught me a few techniques
about foreplay and kissing, it hindered my ability to develop intimacy and meaningful sex in the context of an honest relationship.
Instead, I sought love through sex, was mute in communicating my
needs and desires, got drunk, and fucked men to make myself feel
attractive and desired.

Flat chested and with peach fuzz pubic hair, my childhood sexual experience with a full grown male implanted a fear of what I called naked-hairy-man-body. In high school I didn't have any "normal" relationships with boys. I once took a nice boy whom I liked up to my room and gave him a blowjob while my brother tossed snowballs at my window. Embarrassed and fearful of a relationship, I completely avoided the boy after that. The first person I fucked after Mr. S was the guitar player from Iggy Pop after a concert at the Ritz. I was not yet 17, stoned and on Quaaludes. The guitar player called me back to his dressing room after the show. David Bowie was there, but I was so wasted, his presence barely registered in my consciousness. I walked a few blocks to a dingy apartment in SoHo with the guitar player, who pulled off my clothes, fucked me, and fell asleep on top of me. "Wham! Bam! Thank you Ma'am!" I left the apartment at four o'clock in the morning with my damp underpants stuffed into my purse like rotting leftovers. That was the first of a two-year cascade of meaningless and drunken fucks. The next summer, before I left for college, I went on a sex spree numbed by pot and alcohol or Quaaludes and fucked several guys from the neighborhood. I didn't know how to have a relationship with a man that wasn't based on sex, disembodied and disconnected from emotion, communication, and meaning.

In my senior year in college I had my first real boyfriend, who helped me overcome some of my fears and worries. With him, I had a glimpse of what life could be like in an intimate and meaningful relationship. He was open and communicative, supportive, emotionally generous, and non-judgmental.

On Valentine's Day, after we had been dating for about a year, he asked me if I was afraid of his penis. I was struck dumb by the question. I wouldn't answer it for a long time and I sat beside him in stony silence, wondering how I could admit such a thing. Was I afraid of his penis? Of course I was! It scared the shit out of me. It scared me so much I couldn't even say the word penis out loud. I was afraid of it and his hairy balls. I could not look at his full naked man's body in the light. I had no trouble fucking him or giving him a blowjob (with my eyes closed, of course) but I could not look at it; I regarded it as an alien attached to my boyfriend that I needed to fuck and suck in exchange for love and affection. After I broke down in tears, we talked about this and he helped me make connections between how I thought and felt about sex and my sexual trauma, of which he was aware. That was the first time it registered that I used sex to find and hold on to love, and it took many years of trying and failing at this lesson before it finally stuck.

My husband kisses me. After less than a minute, I pull away.

"You don't like to kiss very much do you?" It's the first time he has asked me about kissing in the 20 years that we've been together.

"It's not that I don't like to kiss, it's that I don't like the way you kiss."

"How do I kiss?"

"You poke your tongue in my mouth and it's stiff. I like a soft tongue."

"Let me try again." He kisses me.

"That's too soft. And don't open your mouth so much."

He kisses me again and after three or four tries, it still doesn't feel right.

"I don't know how to explain it to you."

After a few moments he asks, "Do you remember when we took ballroom dance lessons together before we were married?"

"Yes."

"Maybe it's like that. You couldn't let me lead when we danced. You always wanted to lead me on the dance floor. Maybe we should try that. Maybe I should follow your lead in the kiss."

And just like that, we kiss and he follows the motion of my tongue, and the gentle opening and closing of my lips. And for the first time in 20 years — 20 years! — kissing my husband is pleasurable.

"Wow!" I say. "That was amazing. That was fantastic. Why did it take so long for me to tell you that? Why did it take so long for us to realize that?" It is a sexual epiphany.

My husband is nine years my junior. When we met he did not have much experience in relationships or with sex. He was extremely confident in his knowledge and intellect, but not in his sexuality and attractiveness. He was not threatening and didn't have the Don Juan or Casanova personality that I was typically and obsessively attracted to. I invited him on the first date and made the first move to kiss him in a crowded bar, even though he told me he didn't like public displays of affection. I felt sexually superior and confident. For the first time in my life, my attraction was not rooted in sex nor was it obsessive.

The first 15 years of our marriage were marked by perfunctory sex, usually with the lights turned off. We didn't explore much beyond the conventional missionary and doggy-style positions, with some standard fellatio and cunnilingus thrown in for good measure. In my mind, we "got it over with." And I was perfectly happy with that because it made me feel like I had a "normal" marriage and sex life, whatever I imagined normal to be. I didn't feel threatened by him and sex didn't remind me of my shame. I didn't marry a man who was my greatest sex partner; I married a man I could talk to, spend time with, whom I trusted, and with whom I could build a family. The sex was something I did to secure the meaningful and safe relationship. And I could easily have sex with him even if I didn't really want to because it was quick and routine.

We had vanilla sex until my waning libido made it challenging for me to muster up the energy for what had become a routine fuck every two weeks or so. We rarely talked about our sex life, he didn't know that I had any shameful feelings about it, and I certainly never mentioned that I often had sex with him even when I didn't want to. Or, that in order to reach orgasm I engaged in submission fantasies. Our body language toward each other in bed made it clear that there was frustration (his) and resentment (mine).

One day while walking in the park my husband told me he wanted to have sexual experiences that he'd missed out on in his youth. He was jealous of my sexual experience and wanted to explore a sexual side of himself that he had never expressed: he wanted an open marriage and to seek sex outside our relationship. I was not completely closed to the idea, but it did create a lot of anxiety for me. The topic cracked us open and out spilled words and feelings about our commitment to each other, what an honest relationship is, what sex in the context of our relationship means, how we talk about sex, and how we support each other as life partners.

The conversations we had about sex in the context of an open marriage deepened the understanding of my sexual history and experience, and how it affected our sex life. It led to many "aha!" moments and enabled me to talk about how I felt about sex and why. Through this process I needed to decide if I wanted to have sex outside our marriage, and to untangle what I wanted from what my husband wanted. It was easy to subjugate my needs and desires to his because this is how I had functioned for most of my life. It was never about what pleased me, it was about pleasing someone else; if the other person was happy, I could be happy, or if not happy, then I could certainly deal with the pain or unhappiness for the sake of security in my marriage.

My sexual past also brought to the table issues of submission and domination, power and control, and feelings of shame. One night we were lying in bed. It was clear that he wanted to have sex and I didn't. We had been in this particular dance dozens of times before. He turned to me, looked me in the eye and said, "You don't have to have sex with me if you don't want to. You can say, 'No.'" I buried my head in his chest and started to cry. I spread my naked body across his and just lay there, feeling nurtured and loved and secure. I felt no pressure to have sex even though our naked bodies were pressed against each other. For the first time I felt safe and secure saying "No." Maybe it was because he didn't have an erection, or maybe it was because of all the conversations we'd had up to that point—he knew where I was coming from. I felt protected and safe. I didn't have to have sex with him in order to have his love and affection. To trust and believe that security, to feel it deep in my bones, felt so good.

Later, one morning as he was getting dressed, he said, "You don't look at my body." Instead of shutting down, I realized it was true: I was intimidated looking at his body. Was it because it was hairy and called to mind Mr. S's body? He asked if it would help me to explore his body without any pressure or expectation that we would have sex. He put his hands above his head, did not touch me at all, and let me explore his body in whatever way I wanted. I had the power. Being the one in control felt strange and different and I didn't know how to navigate that at first, but soon I started to like it. The fear and discomfort that I had always felt began to dissolve as I explored his body without an expectation of having to give him anything of myself and without having to pleasure him. That was new; I had always been the one whose body was being explored and probed. I realized I needed to feel comfortable and safe with his body before I was able to take control in our sexual play. I needed to overcome my intimidation of his body and his penis before I could regain my sense of control and pleasure.

Sex feels more playful now, and fun. I look at and wear erotic lingerie, which arouses me and makes me feel incredibly sexy. Sometimes I dress up in sexy costumes and we play out my submission fantasies. I can be overtly submissive by choice rather than by default. I see myself in the mirror wearing a black lace corset and I don't feel ashamed; I'm turned on by my own body and watch myself having sex with my husband in the mirror. Being able to embrace the role of submissive and feel great about doing so is new for me. And I am also exploring the leading and dominant role in our sex play, which makes me feel powerful, sexy, and strong.

My deep need for affection and love as a teenager made me vulnerable to a sexual relationship that was rooted in shame, fear, secrecy, and submission. The process of reflecting on my sexual trauma, opening up old wounds, reading through old journals, and exploring sex outside my marriage has added to the complexity and richness of knowing myself as a sexual human being; it has led to the re-awakening of my sexual spirit. I'm not sure that I can say I have completely restored self-worth and self-esteem. There are days when I still feel shame and embarrassment about sex, but I now have a way to talk about it with the person who is my most intimate and trusted partner. Talking about it gives me power over it. And I feel great!

Teri West is a Harvard Graduate School of Education alumna who has wanted to write about her experiences growing up in the Bronx in the 1970s for the past 35 years and has finally summoned the courage to do so, although on any given day she might be found doubting herself and avoiding her writing, as evidenced by her clean Brooklyn apartment, her two well-fed children, and her invigorating sex life.

As I Am

T. M.

His name was Dominic.

Whenever I talk about him, I feel an almost patholog-ical need to say his name, most likely to make up for the years when I could not.

Everything was very Americana, until you got to the details. It was 1996. I was a 12-year-old nerd suffering from severe depressions. I knew I was attracted to girls. I was also pretty sure that I was a boy despite my "female" body. I had never dated anyone. I was fairly positive no one had ever been attracted to me. I had been out of the closet since 1993, around the same time Brandon Teena was murdered; what I knew of being queer was that it would get me killed. Literally. Liking girls, embracing or even acknowledging the small kernel of myself that longed to be seen as a young man—*those* were the things that were going to kill me, if I didn't get to it first.

Then this huge 16-year-old boy comes out of the shadows. His name is Dominic. We meet under the bleachers after a high school football game. He tells me I am beautiful. He asks me who I am.

He tells me he wants to know me. I know he is too old for me. I know I feel no attraction to him but he is my ticket out. I imagine myself telling the popular girls at my middle school about my high school-football-boyfriend. I imagine the Americana-dream that I have been told over and over I am supposed to want. If I can make myself want it, maybe everything will be OK.

He got my phone number from my older brother. We started talking. We traded pictures, using my brother as the courier. We never spent time together in person because there was no way my parents would let me go out with anyone, much less a 16-year-old young man. And then the violence began.

He started writing raps about me containing terrifying lyrics that coupled sex and violence. He detailed the things he wanted to do to me, the ways he wanted to please me—and hurt me. I told him I did not like it. He told me that he didn't mean it, that they were just lyrics. But he didn't stop. I felt so dirty and so violated. I was terrified.

I didn't realize at that point that the unwelcome sexual words he had been writing to me, about me, for months, that pairing sex and violence as natural, was wrong. I thought I was the thing that was wrong. I had no words to categorize what was happening. We were barely taught about sexual abuse in school, and certainly dirty rap lyrics were never covered in the curriculum. I thought I had no right to have any feelings about it.

My memories get fuzzy around here. All I can remember is fear—fear on so many levels. He was going to hurt me. But also I conceptualized the relationship as what I was supposed to want. This is what a heterosexual relationship was. My options were Dominic, or death by homosexuality.

Instead, I found a third option. I gave up. I broke up with him. I started doing drugs. I started self-mutilating.

About a year later, I got to high school and Dominic and I were in band together. It was our first time seeing each other since the day we'd met under the bleachers. I could tell he was excited to see me. All I remember is terror. And confusion. I wanted escape, however possible. He slipped notes into my locker. I burned them. They all said the same thing: he loved me; I was beautiful; I was his; he would do whatever it took to get me back; he would stop at nothing. And I believed him. He started following me around. He had his friends call me begging me to get back together with him. Two popular girls ambushed me: they didn't understand, they would *love* for someone to care about them as much Dominic cared about me. He was such a great guy. Hidden between the lines was, "Who else is going to love the awkward unpopular nerd?" I told them no. It was like all of the no's I didn't tell Dominic came cascading out of me all at once. I told them no, over and over.

The idea of staying in the same state as Dominic was terrifying, so I ran. My life was a mess, however my grades were still good. At 15, I enrolled in an early college program and moved several states away. And I got better. I quit doing drugs, I found real friends, and I started to learn who I really was.

I also started dating women. I was told I was loved and beautiful, and I believed it. But whenever a relationship got sexual, I took control. I hated being touched and would never achieve orgasm with a partner. I never wanted to feel vulnerable and so I sought out partners who wouldn't mind. I thought this was just part of living in my new "butch" persona. It felt safe. I sought out volatile relationships. I focused my energy on finding chaos. Emotionally, I liked being out of control. But the thing I kept strong control of was my own body. Thanks to Dominic, being touched and violence were linked in my mind; if no one touches me, no one can hurt me.

During my senior year of college, Dominic died in a motorcycle accident. He popped a wheelie and fell off the back. I remember my mother telling me what happened. She thought we had just been friends. She was unaware of his inappropriate and threatened violence in our relationship. She told me what a good boy he had been. I broke my stunned silence to agree. I was sad. I felt broken.

But a small voice told me that what Dominic had done was wrong. Before that moment, I had always thought that I was to blame. I was ashamed. I was fearful that I had ruined a chance at a "normal" life. I still thought there was a normal out there, and I had blown it. It felt like a flood—a sudden awareness that most of what I believed was not true. I didn't know what to do with this new knowledge. It felt like permission to be fucked up. I had been searching for something to blame for my issues. Dominic was a suddenly easy excuse. *Of course* I am prone to volatile relationships. *Of course* my drinking and drug use were a bit excessive. *Of course* I was constantly on the brink of losing myself altogether. *Of course of course of course.*

And then I met Shannon. We were working together at a camp for the summer. I liked her immediately. I felt horrible about this because I had a girlfriend at the time who lived a few states away from the camp, though still in driving distance. We had agreed to stay together as a couple until the end of the summer, and then end our relationship because when camp was over, I was moving to Florida. Meeting Shannon changed that.

I brought a few friends—including Shannon—home to my folks' house for a weekend. I tasked one of them with preventing Shannon and me from sleeping in the same room. She failed. I found myself in my childhood bed while Shannon was camped out on the floor next to me. We talked late into the night. I told her I had a crush on her. She told me that that was very flattering. She told me she liked me too. We fell asleep that night holding hands.

The next week back at camp, we had a night off together. We drove into town and sat in a park by the river. I told her that no matter how much I liked her, I had to be single before I could do anything about it. I told her I could not resist her. She loved all of that. She told me that she respected my need to wait, but added that she didn't have to make it easy for me.

Damn. That was about the sexiest thing I had ever heard from a partner. It felt like a challenge. It made things feel inevitable. Perhaps they were. When we got back to camp that night, she played guitar and sang for me. She was sitting on the bench of a picnic table, and I was sitting behind her with my knees on either side. All my resolve broke. I turned her around, and we kissed.

She and I have spoken about that first kiss several times. We agree it was the single best kiss in either of our lives. Everything was electric. I honestly believe it was the most present moment of my life. I had never felt need like that. I had never felt wanting like that. Sex was something you did once you were in a relationship. It was an act that gave you power. I didn't think that it was about sharing anything with anyone else. Those ideas slipped completely out the window with that kiss. I hiked the mile and a half back to my cabin in the dark with my head aswirl in guilt and bliss and hormones and guilt and guilt and guilt.

Shortly thereafter I dutifully got in the car and broke up with my girlfriend.

A couple of days later the campers were gone for the week, and Shannon and I immediately ran off to find privacy together. We were giggly, nervous, and about to crawl out of our skin with excitement. We had waited so long to be able to touch each other. And when we did, she called me on all of my shit.

She asked me where I was, mentally. She asked me why I was starting in on what was clearly a well-rehearsed and well-guarded sexual routine. She told me to stop. She told me to be in the moment with her. We kissed for hours. We kissed and touched until I began to lose myself in her. She said I had to learn every inch of her body and she had to learn every inch of mine. There would be no "game plan," no "moves."

I didn't like it, at first. It was scary. When she came near my neck, I would recoil. (Dominic had frequently incorporated choking into his lyrics.) Every bit of me wanted to run. But I tried. I learned. We kept practicing. She taught me about my body and about hers.

Our super-sexy summer romance ended, and, without the physical contact, our relationship fell apart. She moved back to Canada, and I moved on to Florida.

That year in Florida was the worst year of my life. I made some bad choices. I let people down—most notably, myself.

If I took one thing away from my time in Florida, though, it was a reevaluation of men. Prior to that year, I had attended a women's college and worked at an all-girls camp. My only interactions with men were with my professors and my family. This was incredibly intentional: men were bad. Men hurt me. Men were all Dominic. And in Florida, I had male co-workers, male neighbors, and male students. One young man, in particular, was incredibly insightful. During our first hurricane evacuation together, we were sitting in the dark (as one does when the power is out). He said, "I know you are a lesbian, but you don't much like guys at all, do you?" I blustered about how false that was. He said he could tell I had been hurt. He told me that he wanted to show me that men could be OK. He spent the rest of the year taking me on friend dates. He would surprise me with flowers. He never made any kind of sexual advance toward me. His kindness healed wounds. I learned to feel safe around him. He was gentle and an amazing friend. He got other nice guys in on his campaign, too. By the end of the year, I had a bevy of outstanding, kind, compassionate, and loyal male friends who wanted nothing more than to show me that not all men were awful, that men could be good.

The next summer, Shannon and I were back at camp, though now we were barely on speaking terms. Things were further complicated by the fact that I was now technically her boss. One of the other directors knew about our past, and to test me, she made me write Shannon up in the first week, just to make sure I would if it was needed. After that, I was pretty sure Shannon would never speak to me again.

Then, Harry Potter intervened. One of the books had just come out. For some reason, Shannon was camped out in the bunk next to mine and we were both reading voraciously on an afternoon off. Gradually, we drifted toward each other. Slowly, over the hours, hands wandered, bodies moved closer. I boldly moved the bunks together. She didn't recoil. She didn't leave. Without saying a word, we were suddenly back together.

We melted together. I had never had sex as intimately as we did that summer. This was the first time I hadn't been consumed with what I was getting or what I was taking away from the experience of being sexual. I remember thinking that, in that moment, I could be more than a collection of the things I had done wrong and the things that had been done wrong to me. My past did not need to define me.

The rest of the summer was intense. Something about the year apart, the missing her, the barely getting started the year before… I was ready. I embraced starting over. Our relationship continued over the year beyond camp. We lived in different cities but visited each other frequently. I learned to love how much she loved pleasing me. The intensity of our touch also came with a degree of emotional chaos, and sometimes I would shut down and go to a dark place. She was always there to pull me out with grace and care.

Of course we did not work out. On the eve of moving across the country to be with her, we called it off. We were both so young, but mostly, she was still too free for me. Our lives were not designed to fit together in the way that our bodies were. And despite all the strides I had made, there were still pieces of myself I needed to reconcile before I could commit to anyone else.

I got sober and I was single for a year. That was the longest time I had been single since my first post-Dominic relationship. I did a lot of healing and a lot of putting away of what I thought I knew about myself.

In time, I met an amazing woman, and I got married. I was able to carry all the things I had learned about myself, about intimacy, and about touch into our relationship. I no longer worried that Dominic would appear around any corner and I no longer carried

the constant fear I had with Shannon that things could implode at
any moment. There is an intimacy that comes with shared chaos;
but there is also an intimacy that comes with calm. In that calm, I
was able to see where the rocky bits remained. The inauthentic part
of me became clear.

I had to admit to myself what I had first realized and pushed
away when I was 14: I was a boy. I was transgender. My body did
not match who I was.

I had been so scared of this truth. For one thing, I had been
taught repeatedly that being a woman was the most amazing thing
about me. Camp and college—these all-female spaces celebrated my
womanhood in a way that made me feel strong, and I had needed
that strength after Dominic. I also carried an ingrained belief that
accepting my manhood meant accepting that I was capable of the
violence and depravity that Dominic had shown toward me. I didn't
want to be what he was. It didn't matter that there were good men
and that I could be one. It didn't matter that plenty of women have
violent and depraved tendencies. Being a man, I thought, made me
capable of the worst.

I needed to eradicate the last barrier between the world and me.
I needed to come to the world from a place of honesty. So I came
out. I started living as a man. And I learned through that process
that *I* get to choose the kind of man I am. I get to build myself the
way I want.

Living an authentic life is about as far away as possible from
the secrets and sneaking around that Dominic chose. Among many
things that therapy helped me to accept is that what Dominic did
was wrong. No caveats. Not my fault. I don't think he was a pedo-
phile. I don't think he was a rapist. I think he was a young man who

was conditioned by popular culture to connect sex and violence. I hope that my silence, my never turning him in, my never telling anyone, didn't enable his journey along a dark path. Even so, I can finally shed the last bit of guilt—it wasn't my fault. I was 12 and 13 when everything happened. I can forgive my silence. And I can speak up now.

T. M. is an activist, artist, and educator living in the Southern United States. He has an amazing wife and a fantastic 17-year-old adopted foster son. T. M. spends his time working with queer youth, hanging out with his family and dogs, and celebrating everyday acts of kindness.

FIND YOUR VOICE AND CARRY A BIG SIGN

Maureen Shaw

At 15, I became a statistic.

In hindsight, the assault itself—committed by someone I trusted—was but a flyspeck on my life's timeline. It was terrifying, but it was finite. Conversely, the prolonged emotional aftermath of the attack has shaped the trajectory of my life.

I did not speak a word of my rape for seven years. Seven long years. Like many victims, I blamed myself and internalized the trauma, which manifested itself in a litany of self-destructive behaviors. It wasn't until my senior year of college that I spilled my secret to a supportive group of students in my women's studies class. It was like a dam burst; once I spoke my truth, there was no going back.

I began attending group therapy for survivors on campus, I spoke at my university's Take Back The Night, and I decided to "come out" as a rape survivor to my immediate family and close friends. I use that term to describe my disclosure because in many ways, I had been living a secret life in which a formative experience—and large part of who I am—was compartmentalized and shelved away. I feared how my loved ones would react upon learning I had been raped. Would they blame me? Be angry that I hid this secret for so long? Think of me as "damaged goods?"

I will never forget the day I told my parents their youngest child had been a victim of rape. The anguish on their faces belied their attempt to be strong, which simultaneously broke my heart and infuriated me; it was the first time I truly grasped the ripple effect of sexual assault. I was angry that my rapist had not only stolen my joy, but had shattered the peace in my parents' hearts. While I had suffered the physical trauma alone, the emotional trauma was now a shared experience.

My parents swallowed their pain to rally around me, as did my siblings and friends once I told them. With each retelling, I realized the shame I had been carrying for so long did not belong to me; it was my rapist's. What's more, I understood that the displaced shame thrived on my silence, and I refused to be complicit in my suffering any longer. For me, that meant dismantling the stigma and humiliation surrounding sexual assault by speaking about it.

Once I began sharing my story—initially among my inner circles and later, more widely as an activist and writer—I found my strength. I felt empowered each time I identified as a rape survivor because I had survived. I waded through some of the ugliest feelings I've experienced to date and I survived those, too.

The more I spoke and wrote about my assault, the easier it was to revisit that dark chapter in my life. And the more I opened up, the more other survivors began to share their stories with me. Slowly, the event that had left me isolated throughout my adolescence transformed into a unifying experience that gave me a sense of community.

Really, community is what propelled me toward healing and gave me the courage to begin advocating for other survivors. I joined the local chapter of a national feminist organization and poured my energy into seeking justice for rape victims. This process came with a steep learning curve, not just about the complexities of sexual assault, but also about myself.

I was a complete rookie when I began volunteering. I was naïve about the systematic and institutional nature of victim blaming and I had no hands-on activist experience. I had zero insight into how different identities can influence a survivor's experience. I was a middle-class, young, white woman and the obstacles I encountered during my healing journey are assuredly different from those facing women of color, men, low income, LGBT, or non-gender conforming/queer people. Consciousness would come with time.

I vividly recall my first protest. Various organizations and individuals came together in outrage over a subpar sentencing recommendation for a convicted rapist. Armed with a sign demanding our justice system take rape seriously, I marched in front of the court alongside veteran activists, and every time I tried to join in the chants ("If you do the crime, you must do the time!"), I choked up.

That lump in my throat wasn't borne out of sadness, but from an overwhelming feeling of togetherness and pride. I was incredibly proud to be part of a movement that dedicated itself to protecting and promoting women's rights, one that fearlessly advocated for sexual assault victims.

Feelings of awe aside, I remained unconvinced of what end result, if any, our action would have that day. As it turns out, our protest and an online petition made a difference; the judge handed down the maximum sentence.

That triumph—my first real taste of feminist activism—taught me a powerful lesson I'll never forget: that speaking up can make a tangible difference. And not just in one's own healing journey, but in the lives of others. I loved playing a part, no matter how small, in that process. Over the course of the next several years, each time I attended a protest, led a group of volunteers in letter-writing campaigns, or sat in a courtroom in solidarity with a victim plaintiff, I shattered the silence that had trapped me for so long. I grew confident, I developed a purpose, and I became fierce.

An unexpected and very welcome sidebar to my immersion in feminism was the reclaiming of my sexuality—on my terms. For years, sex had been transactional, as something I engaged in though never valued, mostly because it felt tainted by my rape. My feminist awakening sparked a sensual awakening. The confidence and strength I drew from activism—in addition to internalizing the feminist movement's emphasis on bodily autonomy—translated to a healthier sense of self: mind and body. Once I learned to believe in myself as a capable, spirited human being with valid feelings and passions, it spilled over to the physical. I respected my body and knew I deserved sexual intimacy.

I have no doubts that feminism helped create the best version of myself. And this is the person my (now) husband fell in love with.

By the time we met, I'd had years of being publicly identified as a survivor and I no longer felt ashamed. Even so, coming out to him in the beginning stages of our dating was decidedly daunting. For the first time in my adult life I was ready and willing to trust another human being on a deeply intimate level, and I was terrified my disclosure would jeopardize our budding relationship. It wasn't rational, it was visceral: It felt eerily similar to the moments immediately before telling my parents.

My fears were (once again) unfounded. He listened empathetically and I was reminded of the cathartic power of sharing my story. As we navigated an emotional and physical relationship over the coming weeks and months, he was patient and followed my lead. It was refreshing to be involved with a person who respected me so much, and his compassion was (is) bottomless. He understands that my rape is a part of my history; it doesn't count against me and it doesn't define me, but it does impact the way I approach life.

As it turns out, it also affects the way I parent. My husband and I have two young children—a preschool-aged daughter and an infant son—and although they're too young to understand the concept of sexual assault, let alone talk about it, we've already begun teaching consent in age-appropriate ways.

Consent is a two-way street, however. As vital as it is for our kids to know they shouldn't be touched without consent, they also need to understand and respect others' physical boundaries. We talk about this regularly with our daughter and plan to do the same with our son as he grows up. I firmly believe that the earlier we help our children establish bodily autonomy, the better.

Now in my mid-30s, in a loving relationship and a mother of two, I've come a long way from the teenager who lived in fear and was well versed in self-loathing, thanks to my empowering trifecta of self-disclosure, feminism, and a supportive partner. I'm proud of who I am today and love myself deeply not in spite of my rape, but because I triumphed over it. It has been a learning process about my own strengths and power, and an inspirational jumping-off point on many occasions. The value of speaking up can't be overstated especially in the face of adversity. I encourage anyone suffering in silence to develop their voice with confidence. It helps to carry a big sign.

Maureen Shaw is a feminist, writer, and proud mama of two. Her writing has appeared widely online, including sherights.com *(which she founded in 2011),* Quartz, The Atlantic, Huffington Post, Mic, Women Under Siege, FeminISting, Fem2.0, Jezebel, *and more. Maureen holds a Master of Arts degree in Human Rights from Columbia University and can't imagine life without feminism or chocolate.*

LIKE A VIRGIN

JUSTINE LARK

There was no religion in my family, no ability to reach out for it, no way through to an understanding of how to deal with life's complexities, and no opportunity to follow a faith in order to find forgiveness. I didn't care. I liked my body and my body knew that the feelings I had were real and exciting. I was sure that touch led to something ecstatic, if not exactly speaking in tongues, then tongue-related. And it did.

I was 14 and I was turned on, full of expectations and desires. I really was. We were in the same class at school; he paid attention to me and smiled a lot. He was kinda tough and kinda shy with brown hair and freckles. We started going out together, meeting on the corner and finding places to make out. It was exciting and we both loved it. I felt no shame. There was nothing that would change my mind about it. I was having sex with my boyfriend; it was 1963.

We were doing it every day at his family's apartment because his mom worked and we could hang out on her big double bed. Sometimes we'd go to my family's apartment, but I was always anxious that we'd get caught there. In the beginning there was no pressure, no abuse, and for about six months it was pleasurable, so thrilling and so consuming. I'm not sure why I changed my mind. I might have gotten worried that wanting sex so much was wrong. More likely I was scared, not of him but for my reputation. I wasn't worried about getting pregnant—though we never used birth control. I was afraid for my *reputation*—yes, the logic was flawed—and when I didn't want to have sex anymore, he used that fear against me. This is when I saw my boyfriend start to change, and I witnessed the beginnings of what that young man would turn out to be.

That bad-boy boyfriend is in jail now… for life…for murder. I had a thing for the bad boys back then. I wasn't worried about my safety; I knew there were people who had my back. But it would take just a few words to kill my reputation.

Back then all we had was our reputation.

The sexual trauma I experienced didn't start out as physical abuse or violence: It was in being controlled. He wouldn't hurt me but he held my reputation over my head to keep me doing things that I used to do and enjoy but I didn't want to do any more, until I reached a point where I couldn't stand it, the fear, the worry about the nasty words that would be said, about my parents finding out. I couldn't go on.

There was nothing available to me. No one could help me. There were no adults, no social workers, no therapists, no counsel-

ors, and the last thing I could do was to tell a friend because if I did,
I'd be known as a slut and a whore. That I managed to get out of this
situation says more about me and not the time. It is what makes me
as strong as I am today. It's why, even with all my little cracks and
insecurities, I know I will always make it. I had to rely on myself. It
was me or nobody.

What I did was start talking. To myself. After a good deal of
talking, I decided it was God I was talking to. I talked to him a lot.
And I made him a deal.

*If you get me out of this, I promise not to have intercourse ever again
until I get married.*

I was able to get out of the relationship with my reputation
intact, and I made good on my promise. I didn't have intercourse
again until I was married. So maybe there's a God after all.

In the meantime I had lots of orgasms, lots of sex, but never
intercourse.

The first person I ever spoke to about my deal with "God"
was the young man I was going to marry, and I did so after we
were engaged. Before the wedding, someone said I needed to see a
gynecologist. The reason for that is unclear but I went and tried to
be a virgin. The doctor kept saying to me, "Are you telling the truth,
are you a virgin?" *No. I've never had sex.* "Did your boyfriend finger
you?" *No. Never.* The doctor tried ten different ways to ask me the
same thing.

He said, "I'm not so sure. You are not a virgin."

I've never had sex.

I left the office with a Pap smear and a fantastical, magical
remaking as a virgin. I was 20.

After we got married and we tried to have intercourse, I could not. It was too painful and just not possible. I didn't go to a doctor. My husband and I took the first seven months of our marriage to work it out, which is probably why I will always love him. That, and we had two children. He saved my life in lots of ways and being able to have intercourse again was just one of them. My mom was a raging alcoholic, and I needed to get out of Dodge. Here was this gorgeous man who was in love with me and I was in love with him and he was taking me to Chicago. He came with a built-in family that I adored. They were working-class, which is how I'd grown up, and together we laughed our asses off. I loved him and his family deeply—I still do—but at some point I knew I needed more on so many different levels, and we separated. He is a lovely human being and he helped me get to a place of security within myself. I consider him my lifesaver, or perhaps savior. My atheist dad is probably shuddering in the afterlife with these words.

In a convoluted process of ending the marriage, I met an unimportant man and because I didn't care, I let it all go. I was totally in lust and for the first time, I could be fully, sexually free. But the first person who helped me to understand sex as amazing and fun was a boy I met after I'd left the bad boy. I loved dancing and dance contests and I met this guy, Billy. God, I loved him. We never had actual intercourse, I still had my promise to keep, though we had sex every afternoon in his basement. It was fantastic and orgasmic and we discovered every part of each other's body. We both got off on whatever we were doing and he never pressured me. His penis was a part of his body but it didn't rule. I couldn't figure that out. His body was tall and lean, not muscular, with a small frame. He felt more female than male to me, and that felt familiar.

There are so many conversations I've wanted to have with Billy since those days when we were sixteen and so sensually, intensely intimate. I tried to look him up years later and found a phone number for his cousin.

"Hello?"

"Hi, I'm a friend of Billy's from the past. I was hoping you could help me find him."

"Who's calling?"

"Justine."

"Oh. I remember you."

(Silence.)

I guess that was *not* a good thing. She did not help me find Billy.

Justine Lark is a lesbian. She lives a good life, maintains her virginity, and works part-time in security.

CLEARING THE DEBRIS
CAIRO GIRL

I have an optimistic nature and an eye for what could work in any situation—and that's not usually a good thing in a revolution or in a romantic relationship.

While we were suffering from the deliberate use of sexual violence against women as a way to undermine the revolution in Tahrir Square, I received a petition about two women in India who were raped and then hung. I was also following the sexual assault awareness work being done on US college campuses, as part of the Yes All Women campaign. It hit me that sexual violence was not a third world problem or a first world problem.

This is a global issue and it is escalating.

I'm an Egyptian woman who has lived overseas at different times in my life. Now, I live nearer to my family in Cairo. I was married to a man, a long time ago. He was always blaming me for "getting the devil out of him by provoking him" or something to that effect in a rough translation from Arabic. I was always trying to be careful to avoid problems. He had developed a good trick where, after he acted violently with me, he faked a heart attack. The first time I believed him and tried to get a doctor.

The second time I realized it was a trick.

There were more gory details of physical violence that I don't need to share. After beating me up, when he realized he had crossed a line and he didn't know what to do next, he usually tried to have intercourse with me. I don't know if he thought that this was a way of making nice, or if beating me up turned him on, or what. I was completely repulsed by him and did not want him near my body — the body he had just hurt and thrown things at. He would have sex and fall asleep, but I would not sleep at all that night.

One of the things I liked was puzzles and previously he had bought me some puzzles, not very big, maybe 50 pieces each. After his violence and forced intercourse one night, I dumped five or six puzzles on the floor and I sat with the pieces all mixed together, and I decided, "I'm going to figure this out."

And I did.

When I heard the dawn call to prayer and light started to seep through the curtains, I looked at those finished puzzles and I realized there and then, "I will survive this. He is not going to crush my soul."

I figured out the puzzle, literally and figuratively.

When someone undermines you consistently and cuts you off from your friends — the regular profile of an abusive relationship — that person becomes your only source for validation. Instead, they deprive you and blame you for doing this or failing that, and while you try to make it work, society adds more pressure. It was crazy making, but I didn't lose my mind. That was my first big moment of realizing that I am strong.

My family was not very supportive through that time. It is hard for a young Egyptian woman to become a "divorced woman." They couldn't fathom having a divorced daughter. They wanted me to stay married, having no idea how to deal with the alternative.

I understand their worry.

Quite miraculously, I managed to get a divorce without going to court and I left soon after on a scholarship to study in England. I remember one time on campus when I was hanging out with other international students and one of them told me, "You get the best out of people." I started sobbing because all I had heard from the man I married had been, "You get the worst out of me, you get the worst out of me." It was not how I imagined myself, yet how could I know? No one had ever told me otherwise. It was helpful to have friends share some of the good things they saw in me. I was nourished by what they reflected back to me of myself.

My first sexual experience was before I was married, and with somebody I knew. We were studying together one night and he started kissing me. I really enjoyed that part. Then other things happened and I had no control over what followed. I remember thinking: "Is this sex? So that's it? Did he enter me? Am I not a virgin now?" I had no idea!

I was 19 and had considered myself a woman of the world, and still I was so naïve I did not know that what happened constituted sex. I liked the kissing and being touched, feeling warm, feeling appreciated. That was pleasurable, even if the other part was so shocking.

After talking to a girlfriend who also knew him, we were sure he had done this to other girls. I did not know what to do. He called me back a few days later to make nice and it was confusing. He wanted to meet again to study. He was such a sweet talker that I went. I don't remember if we had intercourse or not, but by going back there I thought maybe I was seeking pleasure, or there must have been some joy in it. I don't know, because I blocked what happened that second time at his house. However, I remember the first event very, very clearly: I left his apartment and went down to the street. I started running, and something snapped in my lower back.

Snap, I heard the sound.

Whatever broke in me on a soul level affected me physically. Later, looking back, I thought, "Are you stupid? You put your hand in the fire. Twice." I felt I had returned knowing what could happen and I couldn't forgive myself. I still shudder if I hear the name of that man, or when I walk into that neighborhood, or have to be on that street. And decades later I'm still treating that pain in my back. I am aware of this spot by my inability to move easily on a daily basis, and I continue to treat it medically with physiotherapy and chiropractors. Still, I know that there is more than the doctors can see.

I also know that healing my sexuality is integral to the healing of my back injury and that being with a partner with whom I share a healthy sexual life will support further healing.

I never labeled myself as a "victim" or "survivor." I never, ever, subscribed to that role. It helped that I disappeared for a few years in England. I think that was a way of ignoring the issue—my way of coping. Years later, I was electrocuted in an accident in my apartment. To heal from that, I needed to "rewire" myself. Because

Western medicine was not helping at all, I was receiving a lot of cranial sacral work. During the treatment process my old traumas surfaced. I was able to describe to the woman who was doing the energy work what had happened to me at the age of 19. It was the brain trauma from the electrocution that allowed these memories to surface, nearly 25 years later. When your body is weak, the weak and vulnerable points can become activated by a trauma. It took the healing work I did after that accident for me to realize that what had happened was rape, and to be able to name it as such and start to process it emotionally and spiritually.

Generally, I'm not a slow learner, but I can take my time to process things. Healing is not a push-button. Healing is working through all the issues that created the vacuum to start with. Like my puzzles, I had to figure it out one piece at a time. I began to put it together in a kinder way, to not blame myself, to forgive myself, as well as release that deep emotion I held locked inside. And then I realized: *OK, now you need to forgive them.*

And then I thought: *Assholes? I have to forgive the assholes?*

For me, I was not free until I freed myself from those connections. It took me a couple of years to wrap my head around that. I refused to accept it. After years of resistance, I had to ask myself why I was still recreating the same patterns in other new relationships. Eventually, I understood on a deeper level that I was part of those situations, and that acceptance was so empowering. I've learned to ask myself: "What do I attract on a vibrational level? How can I attract things differently?"

A colleague of mine is constantly writing about harassment, saying, "Cairo is a horrible city right now to walk as a woman, even if you are completely covered with a burka." But she is looking for this kind of behavior to validate her sense of how horrible the world is, and of course she's finding it. Almost every post she puts on Facebook says something terrible: that she has been mugged, or someone broke her camera, or the taxi driver harassed her. I care for her and I'm trying to help her, but what I am telling her about creating her reality does not register with her at all.

"What are you saying? You mean I am making them harass me?"

"Nooooo, but kind of yeeeessss."

If somebody told me this when I was 19, I wouldn't have understood. It wouldn't have been helpful to hear this before I went through my own journey of healing. But understanding this has changed the course of my life in a profound way. Now that I'm older-wiser, I am aware that I'm able to create safe boundaries, to *not* re-create those experiences. I don't get harassed on the streets of Cairo. Yes, sure, I dress in a modest way—I don't wear many things I would have worn in England, for instance—and I do not get any harassment. I do not draw that energy.

To be clear, it is never the victim's fault. I *never* blame somebody who has been assaulted or subjected to violence for creating that violence, nor do I ask, "What was she wearing?"—that kind of sick logic. I defend the right of every woman to wear whatever she wants, to be whatever she wants whenever she wants, but she also needs to find ways to keep herself safe on many levels, not just the physical. I'm talking about manifesting protection, awareness, or strength that can only come from within. It's in the fortifying of one's soul and the making of energetic boundaries.

I am not currently in a sexual or romantic relationship, and that's because my standards are higher than they used to be—and that is a good thing! My standards are higher and I live in a very conservative place and time, and that does not make for a winning combo. But I try. Every few months, I think maybe there is something interesting in this man or that guy. And often there is not, sadly. I scare them off sometimes, and that's also OK.

My relationships at this time are the friendships that I have been lucky to find and to create. It's like a sisterhood of the soul in many ways. Having this community helps with my feeling of connection and also with remembering different parts of myself, the different roles I play, and the adventures I've had. It's wonderful to be supported by beautiful and powerful and strong and fragile women who create my network. This is something precious, something I wish I'd had when I was younger.

I had started attracting this kind of light, this attitude and like-mindedness, before I traveled out of Egypt. I volunteered in feminist organizations and talked to people about women's rights, domestic violence, and similar issues. I fought for the right to work late and I fought for the right to work in my chosen profession. I fought to travel alone. I fought to attend a festival in another town. I fought for my existence. In Egypt, none of what I wanted to do was considered OK.

I went to London to work after I completed my Master's degree. My first day coming out of the Tube, I was handed a magazine at the subway entrance. I was surprised to see that all of the articles completely objectified women. I thought, "I am from a developing country, and here I am in the "civilized" world, and *this* is what women are being told as they get off the Tube —how to dress and look sexy at work?" It was like a conversation from another century. It was shock after shock. I participated in a Zero Tolerance campaign about violence against women and children, and here again, I was hearing similar stories to those I had heard in Egypt. I saw women accepting things they shouldn't, women who blamed drinking—not the guy—for the assault. My first Christmas in England I was at a friend's house and all the women were in the kitchen and all the men were in the other room watching football. That dynamic was the same dynamic I was running away from. And this is when I realized it's not just "us," as in Egyptians; the fight is universal. The women in England need liberation as much as the women in Egypt, and in many cases maybe more so, because many of them are not even aware of the need.

Regarding sexuality, I was self-taught. I read books. I know I seem comfortable in my body and in my sexuality, and yet it's also true that when there's another person in the room, it becomes more complex. For myself, it took a long time to accept that sex is part of a healthy life and healthy body, and to fully enjoy being in my body. I was thinking about this in bed this morning, as I was engaging in my "extracurricular activities." (By the way, every woman should have a very good vibrator. I highly recommend it.)

I have struggled with an excessive desire to please others, limiting the space for my pleasure. "I don't matter that much," is how I was conditioned with sex early on. Later with lovers, I would be so careful that they had an enjoyable experience, and my needs and my desires were not a part of the experience. I used to think it was just me who felt this way, and I've learned this isn't true. There are so many women with an amazing capacity for joy, and they can enjoy themselves in their body and have a fantastic series of undulating big O's and small o's...and then there's a sexual partner involved, and, "*What*? He gets tired of *what*? He doesn't want to do *what*?" It's very frustrating!

Enjoying my body is both about sexuality and sensuality. Finding sensuality has meant being open to experimenting, and through time, trial, and error, to finding my boundaries. I am a physical person. I do lots of yoga and trained in body work, so I regularly deal with being in the body, touching the body, and healing others. I enjoy giving energy work as much as receiving it. It's a way of connecting to the body and understanding its inherent ability for joy that we all presumably have. At times I've thought, "OK, maybe I'm sensual, but not sexual," and then I realized, "No, I am both sensual and sexual. I'm just with the wrong *person*!" I need a partner who is aware, sensitive, and comfortable with themselves, and is also comfortable with me being a strong woman who knows what I want, and how I want to enjoy myself and my sexuality. I want someone who will appreciate the gift of me sharing pleasure in my body. If we are both having a sexual experience, we should both have sexual pleasure. I think of this as a basic human right. The Declaration of Human Rights does not have this as an Article, but it should! Eventually, after many years of being small or invisible, or not acknowledged, or not claiming my space in a relationship, I trusted the voice within and I've started to allow for this possibility.

While I didn't have a mentor in learning about my sexuality, I have become other people's mentors—people I work with, especially young women I know who are getting married and have no idea what to expect. Sexuality in Egyptian culture, as within many others, is such a taboo. I am able to share what I have gone through, not in the details about this specific event or that particular pain, but enough to provide gravitas when I talk with people who are going through troubled times or physical ailments. I can let them know that this time shall pass, and that it's possible to come out of their situation and enjoy life as beautiful powerful women.

When I was returning to Egypt after living overseas for a number of years, I bought a few books on sexual education for children and young adults. When my nephew turned sixteen I said to my sister, "I have these books for the kids. Which one is right for his age?"

I think she was mortified.

I didn't want to interfere with her parenting, so I just gave her the books so she could decide what she wants to share with her kids and when. She has since told me she had my nephew read a chapter or two, and she keeps the books hidden. I don't know if I will ever be allowed to have conversations about sex with my nieces and nephews. I don't want them to go through any of the pain or challenging experiences I have, and I wonder if there is a way to help them find their power, to connect to a bigger source in themselves so they are never victimized.

Talking about my journey to a happy and healthy sexuality has been much easier than I thought it would be. I thought it would be opening wounds, but I feel good. I feel it's empowering to talk about this. A couple of stories came to mind that I would not want to see in print. But the process led me to wonder if it was time to revisit these things and clear out more debris. I have since talked about them, not because of the pain, but because in talking I have transcended these events and overcome the pain.

One of my colleagues is a tough woman, a force to be reckoned with. One day she told me, "You are the strongest woman I know." That gave me chills. It still does when I think of it. I don't raise my voice. I don't fit the stereotypical image of strong. But I'm tough. In many ways, I'm grateful for all that has happened to me. Sometimes I imagine if I had married a nice guy, I would never know I was such a strong woman.

My friends say that is not true. I would be a strong woman because I *am* a strong woman.

When I was in India a couple of years ago, I was buying scarves and I saw a beautiful one and thought, "I will give this to my partner, when I meet him. It will be my gift to him, a gift I found before we met each other." Every now and then I wear it because I like the energy of feeling I'm connecting to him.

And, "If I never meet the partner," I've told myself, "I get to keep the lovely scarf."

Now I am thinking I really like the scarf. I have second thoughts about this partner coming to take it.

I might go to India and buy ten more, just in case.

Cairo Girl tries to enjoy life's rollercoaster journey and make the most out of every experience. She loves music, flowers, and yoga. Cairo Girl thrives when she's near water, trees, and evolved people and is eager to share joy and great stories with the world.

ALONE WITH MY BLISS

KYLE D. ANDREWS

I'm a surviving thriver in mid-recovery. I know that this will always be a part of my life. It's part of who I am, the good parts and the bad parts.

I am using this writing to repair the setbacks that have happened. It's a pleasant win-win, an actual in-the-moment-of-healing thought.

Recovery is like a puzzle, discouraging though alluring at first. As time goes on, and with practice, I can complete some sections of the puzzle without hesitation. With other sections, I must not get discouraged, and remind myself it's normal to have obstacles, and that's not a reason to give up. There's no Little Orphan Annie's Secret Decoder ring. I have to make my own ring so when a situation arises, either negative or positive, with a friend, family member, stranger, or the one I love, I can communicate clearly. It takes practice. The old me would try, fail, and say, "Screw this, it's hopeless." As a person who's always in a hurry, I still have to work on patience.

As a gay man who is a survivor, sexuality for me has been confusing and difficult. Identifying that what happened was wrong, was difficult. Maybe those who abused me thought I was gay and that's why they picked me?

Nope. I was prepubescent, broken, and an easy target. PERIOD.

Most of my intimate relationships have been based solely on sex, though the ones that included other shared interests lasted longer. Sex used to be performance. I'd give my partner-du-jour what I thought he wanted, and I did it well. I was called a stud. Told that I was the hottest sex EVER. Once it was over, I could never get out of there fast enough. I'd have sex outside our relationship because I didn't associate sex with love. I didn't want to let my guard down and be vulnerable.

At some point, I had a partner living with me for six months, and while I was packing his lunch one day, I saw his meds in his workbag, accidentally finding out he had HIV. We were not using protection. This flipped in me a switch of nihilistic dysfunction. I thought if I got HIV, it was what I deserved. Eventually he moved out, I continued to have high risk sex, and I was diagnosed with HIV.

As time marched on, my perception of love, sex, and relationships remained distorted. I was having lots of sex but it was never fulfilling. I was introduced to crack and meth—WAHOOO! Now it was "fun" to have unprotected sex with many people at once while doing hard drugs. I thought, "Well, I got the AIDS, what else could go wrong?" What went wrong was not just sexual relations, but also my health, work, family, and friends. It all crumbled around me.

I contracted Hep-C and my mental and physical health spiraled out of control. I picked up several diseases and developed full-blown AIDS, with sores all over my body. I was still using drugs. Losing my job forced me to sell my house. I rented for a bit and spent rent money on drugs. I wanted to die and almost did. Eviction left me homeless. I had no friends or a place to go from all the destructive behaviors that stemmed from not just drugs, but through misconceptions of what a real, true friend is. My first lover and his housemate took me in. They had a couple of house rules: no crack and to only smoke pot in the garage. This was my turning point, my decision to make a change about drug use—although I still didn't know why I was an addict. I knew I had issues but I didn't know the root cause.

Prior to getting into recovery, I met a wonderful man named Jim Henry. He lived far away but we chatted online over many years. He was willing to talk with me when I was still active with drugs and he did his best to help me. He was a soul mate. As our friendship blossomed, we became lovers. He did everything in his power to assist me in every way I needed: with physical issues, HIV, chronic pain, and Crohn's disease. He loved me so much.

One night, after a long time apart, we were having a romantic candlelit evening. He stepped out to freshen up, and when he returned to be with me, I destroyed the mood by saying, "Let's go, let's do it—hurry up." Stunned, he jumped back and said, "What the fuck did they do to you?" I was hurt; so was he. I didn't know what I'd done wrong. It was at this point he began to sense something big had happened to me in childhood, which in turn led to me recognizing that I had been sexually abused.

Years later, at a retreat called Paths of Courage, I realized that so much miscommunication came from my lack of knowing how to love and have sex with people I love. That's what had happened

with Jim. He and I were able to talk about it when I got on the therapy train. In therapy, I began to recall other lovers in my history and
understand why I had chosen them: some because they were very
sexual, some because they were romantic. I recalled one who was so
caring and giving to me I ran off, because I was uncomfortable. I'm
sure some could have lasted the test of time if I met them now.

Whether it was excessive drinking, doing street drugs, fighting,
stealing, hurting others, attempting suicide, or neglecting my own
needs, they were all side effects of trauma. I started the healing journey in 2007 by stopping daily street drug use. After a brief relapse
in 2012, I got into The Fred Victor Centre for Addiction and found
a doctor who saw me not as an addict, but someone who had been
abused as a child and was coping via drug use.

Finding Dr. Young was a turning point. We got along well and
he stuck with me. True grit, I would say. He's done a world of good
by helping me to identify triggers, both good and bad, and to discover the best coping skills to use when triggered. He didn't judge
me for using medical cannabis, which was for complications with
HIV medications; he even understood my addiction to painkillers,
prescribed for me after an injury. He gave me the slack and a strate-
gic push to give them up on my terms.

Dr. Young also referred me to a sexual abuse recovery program.
I did not want to do the group thing. I believed my abuse history
wasn't significant enough to warrant being in the group. And, what
if my being gay made the other men uncomfortable?

What if, what if.

Dr. Young assured me it would be beneficial, despite my concerns. I went. It was quite uncomfortable. Nevertheless the men wel-
comed me, attesting that they dealt with the same emotions when

they joined the group, and that over time the group would become a safe space to sort through the chaos.

I discovered that regardless if it was one time or a hundred, sexual abuse damages us all. I learned about their relationships with family, friends, and lovers: similar to mine, yet different. I learned I preferred sex that's associated with love; that for me, casual sex, which I had thought was good, wasn't good for my spirit. If our brains are hot for each other, then my body can get hot for your body. It means I like to have food before I get nude. As this journey goes on, I've become more and more uncomfortable with random sex with strangers. I no longer plan to take unavailable men or lovers out of desperation because when it's over, I'm alone with my dog, and my emotional and spiritual needs haven't been met. My judgment has changed. Being vulnerable means getting hurt occasionally. Like the lotto, I've got to be in it to win it.

I got deeper into recovery, and it became more and more difficult to perform as a people-pleaser in the sack. I wanted to be pleased and satisfied, too. I too wanted to snuggle and spend the night or the day together. I feel my reason for being a people-pleaser, not just with lovers but also with friendships, was that I was desperate to be in a relationship even if I didn't know how to be OK with it happening, and even if I received nothing in return. My past behaviors drew in all kinds: some were great, like my first lover and Jim, others not so much. Many damaged or scarred me, perhaps not on purpose, but because I allowed it; the results left everyone feeling used and unloved. We were drawn to each other out of dysfunction. I discovered the man who hid his HIV status from me had been raped in his 20s by a man with AIDS who transmitted it to him.

I've learned that there's more to life than just sex and/or love. Those things could happen at any moment, but if I'm not happy when I find them, finding them won't make me happy. I know that now. I strive to be happy every day, and that can come from something as simple as treating myself to comfort food on a bad day. I'm opening up to spending money on hobbies as part of taking care of myself. For example, I have new confidence with music. I was envious of people who could play music and never ever thought there'd be a day I'd say, "I can play an instrument." (It goes back to a King and Queen pageant in 1988 when Ashley MacIsaac took my crown because he could play the fiddle.) I always thought that people who played an instrument were special. I bought a djembe after playing one in retreat workshop and receiving lots of encouragement. My teacher, Y Josephine, tells me I'm talented and she sees lots of potential.

When I first met Dr. Young, he asked me what my goals were. I told him they were to get a dog and to one day own a house. The dog was possible, the house was out of my reach. He told me to get the dog; I was ready. I wanted a dog because I remembered back to my childhood dog, Cuddles, who comforted me whenever I was going through the emotions of abuse, emotions of feeling alone and not loved. When I began to look for a dog, I wanted one that looked like Cuddles. After months of searching I found Duke online. When I met him, I fell in love with him instantly (even though he barked in my face). I connected to him partly because he had been abused, and partly because he was so loving in spite of being abused.

With Dr. Young's help I got documentation sorted to have Duke as an emotional support animal. We get to fly together. He even gets his own train ticket with his name on it. In a way, getting a dog is what I needed: a purpose, a reason to do something because if I didn't I would die. Last Christmas I had an apartment fire and lost everything, and Dukey helped me cope.

At the core of this healing journey are periods of loneliness. I know that sounds sad, but in a way it's not that bad. Alone time is time to think and to work on me. This journey is a lot of hard work. My group calls me "resilient," and I'd like to add "tenacious," with an animal instinct to survive despite all these roadblocks.

I have to tell you it's not all sunshine, rainbows, and lollipops. I get depressed and down, and I am also happy and up. *C'est la vie!* You can't be happy all the time because how the hell would you know if you were happy or not? There's a gland in the brain called the pineal gland, close to where Buddhists identify the third eye. It's the gland that makes us feel good with dopamine and serotonin. Being sad doesn't produce anything in the brain; only bliss produces these chemicals. I believe everyone can be happy because being sad is just your pineal gland not producing. Learning this helped me because I now know that my brain isn't being flooded with sad chemicals—I'm just dealing with a lack of the happy ones.

PTSD is a brain thing. An anti-drug PSA they used to have here in Canada featured a brain with a bunch of electrical wires. Clippers cut through the wires and the brain began to smoke. The message on the screen was, "Drugs rewire your brain!" For those of us who have coped with both drugs and sexual abuse, even more brain healing and new wiring is required. In science, any electrical pulse has a magnetic inductance, which is similar to an electrical circuit. Our bodies use electrical pulses to send signals to the brain, and these signals negatively affect our brain when we are being abused.

It's as if my brain were an electrical circuit that's been fried, shorting out, as if it was an overloaded circuit board.

It took this journey into recovery to find my faith in my ability to decode things and learn from them, and it has led to a total 180-degree change of attitude and energy; I have started taking better care of myself, listening to my feelings, and finding my bliss. I'm learning that self-care is bliss. I practice with the tools I've been given. I've begun to do things I did when I was the old responsible me, like paying bills on time. Or, the best one is setting everything out for my day: oatmeal in the bowl with a spoon of honey, and tea—I've cut out the sugar. I am fueling my body for this journey, which makes me feel good, and feeling good makes me happy. Like a smile, self-care is contagious. I can take the little joys and roll them up into bigger joys.

Letting go of the anger needs to be done at some point in the journey. I have to remind myself that life is not out to get me or punish me with all this sorrow. Suffering doesn't make me righteous and it isn't why I'm here. And that sucks. It really does. I love being angry. I'm good at it—I can go from zero to 1000 in a second if you say the wrong thing. It pisses me off when people use the word faggot: "I'm a faggot so back the fuck off," was my pre-recorded response.

I believe anger is rooted in my childhood abuse. I want to right a simple wrong. Trouble is, these things happen all day every day. Getting emotional is a waste of my amygdala. I've learned that anger is a waste of energy that is pent up for feeling fucked out of a normal childhood… a normal relationship, normal friends, normal experiences, normal housing, normal everything. What is normal? I try for regular. HIV made me face that. I felt for a long time that I deserved to suffer, as if it were fate. It was comforting and familiar to suffer. That is messed up.

I've corrected some circuits in my brain through a lot of different strategies, and other circuits seem to be auto-correcting. I take control of what I can. I am my own savior. I have no regrets for the decisions I made to cope with the pain. I never asked to be molested. I never wanted to be in pain. It wasn't my fault, so why continue to punish myself?

The truth is my abuser stole my innocence, my trust in others and of authority, and my childhood. Taking back what's rightfully mine means they lose: they lose the power they had over me in the aftermath of the abuse. Setting boundaries gives me back the power they took from me; they can't hurt me any more unless I allow them to. I've learned to recognize when I'm being asked to do a favor for someone that will cost me too much to accommodate them; that's people-pleasing and it mirrors the accommodation that happened in the sexual abuse. And setting boundaries has even included eliminating certain people altogether, even people I love and cherish. I can say no.

Some days I feel like I haven't accomplished much. I look back at the last few years and I know I've come light-years, yet I get discouraged when the process isn't as fast as I'd hoped. As time marches on, I worry that after 14 years of having HIV, I may become too sick or ill to be in love or find a steadier happiness. If I become too sick and can't find love or total happiness, this would all be a waste of time. I ask myself, "Would I rather be in the matrix with fake friends and fake love and unstable emotions or would I rather have a real life with a few but higher quality relationships and activities?" I have my answer. We can't predict the future. There could be a cure for HIV next year. The fears are the old me, echoing old thoughts, because I know anything is possible, including happiness. I can find my bliss.

Kyle D. Andrews was born and raised in a small fishing and lumber village in rural Nova Scotia. He is a former telecommunications analyst and a former homeless addict who now is living on disability in one of the poorest housing projects in Toronto. Recovery led him to the Male Survivor Network and to finding his emotional support pooch. His interests include riding motocross, camping, fishing, kites, beaches, travel, and swimming. He describes himself as a "thriver" and as an aspiring writer, photographer, musician, and artist.

Year of the Make-Out

Told by Tara Abrol

composed by Cathy Plourde

I call this The Year of the Make-Out. I have come to realize I love making out.

Every year on our birthdays, my best friend and I create a list of goals we set for ourselves in accordance to the number of years we are turning; this year it was 32. One of my goals this year was no sexual intercourse. I had realized when it comes to sexual intercourse, fear and doubt and "this" and "that" sometimes pop up. So I decided, *You know what, take that the fuck off the table, have your fun with where you're at, and then, we'll see what happens next year.*

In thinking about sexuality as someone who has dealt with trauma, one of the questions I needed to answer was "What's going well now that you have healed?" Up until recently I still thought I was fucked up. I've been thinking, I don't know, because things are not going well; I don't think I've reached the pinnacle of my healing. My idea of reaching full healing has been that I will now be sexually engaged and active and interested all the time

and I will have no fear or doubt and *blahblahblahblah*. But I haven't
had sex with a man for this entire year. I've wondered what if it's
not perfect when I do have sex again?

My feelings about sexuality come in waves; sometimes I feel
great about it; sometimes I feel I'm such a loser and wonder what I
am going to do. In meditation recently I realized those worries are
total bullshit. The fact that I have taken a year off from sex or that I
could even make that decision for myself lets me know, hell yeah,
I *have* made it. I have accepted where I'm at with my sexuality,
whereas even a short time ago I still had shame around it. I am at
the highest point so far, and that highest point is fully accepting my
sexual self, which happens to include moments of great confidence
and moments of doubt.

Historically, I have battled with the concept of sexuality as
"performance." I used to feel I had to be more sexual or more interested in sex or that my sexuality should look a certain way; basically
I was faking it because I had no sense of my own sexuality. I had
been performing for my entire life. I had never given myself the
opportunity or the self-love to figure out: *What do I like? What do I
want to do? What turns me on?* Even as I hit my 30s I was still fighting
with ideas about what was normal. *When I'm in my 30s, I can't just
make out with someone,* right? *We're not 14 anymore. It has to lead to
sexual intercourse—adult sexuality includes intercourse—* right?

There used to be a lot of "Right?" in my life in relationship to
my sexuality. And I've decided to have no more questions about
normalcy. My sexuality is whatever the fuck I want it to be.

I'd describe my sexuality as shy and curious. Now I can sense
when I'm starting to perform. I can recognize my confusion and
stop to think about it. I still feel confused at times but I'm much

more at ease with who I am as a sexual being. The more honestly people can talk about what is actually going on in their sex lives, the more stable and satisfied we'll all be.

Writing this piece is a part of my journey, as is the fact that I've based my entire career around sexuality education. I became a sex educator because I'd had absolutely no sex education. My dad immigrated to the US from the foothills of the Himalayas in Jammu, India, in the 1970s and my mom was born and raised in Brooklyn, New York as a strict Italian-Catholic. (I like to say that the only two things their cultures have in common are a love of food and a refusal to ever discuss sex.) We moved around a lot before I went to a high school in Georgia that was primarily conservative and Christian, and the Sex Ed sucked. Sexuality was in my face all the time and I had no idea what I was doing; unfortunately, I experienced a lot of trauma because of my lack of education and awareness. No one ever talked to me about sex. Ever.

People—especially other young people I was talking to—would spout a lot of bullshit about sex, and I would spout a lot of bullshit about sex, and we all talked about sex like it was the best thing ever. But that was not my experience of sex. My experience of sex was that it was painful, scary, and *nothing* like what everyone said it was. As I got older, I began to sort out the bullshit. I started asking my friends a lot more questions, particularly around what was normal. "What's so great about sex?" "How often do you have an orgasm?" "In what position is it easiest for you to have an orgasm?" I asked questions because I thought, *Shit, if your sex life is this great, come on and help a sister out!*

I used to believe that I didn't know what was going on, that I'd never get there, that I'd be doomed to be confused and doomed to keep up the façade. I've grown up with the idea that bad things happen, that's life; so shut the fuck up. I never told anyone about my sexual trauma. I knew some hard shit had happened to me and there were chunks of memories that were "unfortunate" and should stay as buried as possible. I had internalized the "unfortunate" incidents; the need for alcohol during most of my sexual encounters had become normal, and any underlying feelings of discomfort around sexuality were shameful and abnormal. Everything was my fault. I had not made the connection of my fear of sexual intercourse to my trauma.

As a therapist and a sex educator, I talk honestly to young people about sex and I encourage them to talk honestly with each other. I am also creating more conversation among adults about sex. Many adults are confused about their sexual lives because they, too, received terrible-to-no sex education or have experienced trauma themselves. Sexuality is much more than the penis entering the vagina or the tongue licking the (fill in the blank). It is more than pregnancy and STI prevention. Sexuality education includes talking about relationships, communication, gender, and emotions. We commit a disservice to young people when we leave them stranded to figure out one of the most complicated aspects of the human experience by themselves, and, as was true in my case, this lack of education can have serious, dangerous, long-lasting effects. Sexuality is intimately linked to our personal development, and yet shame is forced upon us for any number of reasons.

Looking back, I believe part of why I accepted my sexual trauma as normal was directly related to the fact that my dad hit me as a young person. Because my dad was physically forceful and disrespectful of my body when I was a child, such mistreatment figured into what I accepted from men when I became a teenage girl. I grew up thinking it was normal for my father to grab me by the hair or push me around, so when other men behaved similarly or worse, I didn't question it. I wish parents would recognize that from the minute a child is born, all the ways they are treated affect them and their expectations of how they will be treated by others.

Growing up, I greatly relied on my mother. There was never any doubt in my mind that she loved me and was there for me. We have a tight relationship, and I appreciate that we are both now able to view each other as adult women. When I was younger and didn't yet have my own perspectives, my mother's beliefs and the church's teachings (martyrdom, the perspective that horrible things make you stronger, or that there's a reason for everything) motivated me and shaped me into the person I am; however, now I find those beliefs and practices detrimental. I never fully embraced Catholicism and there were many years I didn't know what I believed; at some point—I'm sure many things led up to it—I connected with God as a feminine being. That connection allowed me to embrace my own feminine divine and has become central to my spiritual beliefs: the divine spirit lives within all of us.

Getting to know for myself what sexy or sensual looked like took time. I had a lot of doubt in my physical body, and I've had health issues because of it. I think this is from the trauma I carried for years before I found the confidence to deal with it. I'm a dancer, so figuring out what I personally, in my soul, feel is sexy has been achieved through movement, by being in my body, and by loving it. I have much more energy and light than I did before I came into my sexuality. I call it "owning my sexy," which was one of my birthday goals a few years ago, and now, *please*, that's *how* I live my life! To own my sexy has been amazing and empowering. It lets me determine for myself what is sexy and understand how that changes over time.

Getting my sexy on can mean so many different things! Sometimes it's just me in my gym clothes; sometimes it's about dressing up. But it's not only about clothes; it's about relating to my physical body. I like to strut down the street, I like to move like a woman, I like to accentuate my curves, and I like to *be* in my body. When I am connected to my body, I feel a connection to who I am on a spiritual level. This is recent for me. My sexy also comes from the inside; it's not that external, performed sexuality from back in college when I had to wear an outfit that was "sexy" in order to feel sexy.

I joined a peer-counseling group when I was in my mid 20s and stayed with that for about five years. The therapy was based on mental health counseling theory, going after the trauma, processing the feelings, and then reframing the story. When I started the mental health work, recognizing myself as a victim was really, truly empowering. I started to realize I had been victimized in multiple ways and suddenly I wondered if I'd spent my whole life being a victim to men. That was difficult. Prior to this counseling experience, I never would have considered myself a victim.

At first it was empowering for me to know that sexual trauma is a terrible thing that happened, that it should be recognized; I should talk about it and I shouldn't feel shameful or embarrassed. After a time (years) I started getting to a point where I felt I was OK, and it felt as though I was just retelling my trauma stories over and over. I was becoming overly identified with those stories and I was never going to be able to move forward if I couldn't figure how to accept my victimization without over-identifying with it. To be honest I had no idea where to go from there.

At that point, I didn't use the term "survivor" because I didn't feel like I had survived much of anything; I felt like my whole life was in shambles and had always been in shambles. I was a hot mess and couldn't get my shit together. I had never realized why. Then, I was able to connect my shambles to being repeatedly victimized.

OK, now what? Still in shambles here.

As I came to understand my own trauma more, I began to feel more empowered. I started telling men I was in relationships with about my trauma. Every single time I did this, it turned out horribly. At the time, I blamed these men for how badly it went. I still believe they bear the brunt of the responsibility for being completely inept at handling it, but I've realized the reason I was telling these men about my trauma: I was seeking healing. Subconsciously, I was thinking, *I'm going to tell this man I was raped, I'm going to cry, he's going to hold me, he's going to tell me "I'm so sorry that happened to you, it never should have happened."*

You know, what I'd wanted to hear my whole life.

No surprise, I never got that response, yet I kept trying over and over and over, cycling through the pattern: Each new man would be terrified and awkward and would have no idea what to do and would leave and I would feel like I was damaged goods.

In retrospect, I understand what I was going after, and realize that by no means was I ever going to find it that way. I needed to do the real healing for myself on the inside; I was never going to find that through anything people did on the outside. I needed to internally hold and love myself and let parts of myself grieve for as long as necessary. This is what *I* needed to do; I won't say what other people need, because we all heal in our own particular and personal ways.

For most of my sexual life, I wasn't making conscious decisions around my sexuality at all. I felt disempowered and fearful, which I didn't want to admit. I also felt pressure—pressure to be sexual. External messages on that were clear. Otherwise you're a weirdo, you're abnormal, you'll never be in a good relationship, people will not love you, there is something wrong with you, et cetera. In order to balance my sexuality with this pressure I consumed alcohol, or I convinced myself that the relationship was further along than it was. I'd tell myself and others, "Yeah, we're totally in love." It was a lot of me lying to myself.

I call this the Year of the Make Out, because to be clear, I am sexual with people; I'm just not having sexual *intercourse*. That's where my trauma lived. Intercourse was scary and painful. I chose to have a year of no intercourse as a birthday goal because, even though there have been periods in my life when I didn't have sex, whenever I have met someone I've gotten involved very quickly. I've rushed ahead of the feelings. I would have to rush headlong into sex because I had to beat all the feelings of fear, mistrust, and self-doubt. The pattern became: the first year was great; the second year I'd hit a wall when all of the stuffed feelings caught up with me—I'd be totally disconnected and stop wanting to have sex; and then we would break up. That's what my sex life used to look like. So for this year, I am engaging in sexual behavior, except inter-course, and I'm finding it easier to not feel trapped by my feelings.

Getting here has been a lifelong thing. I believe in synchronic-ity; many little bits and pieces and people brought me to this place. Around the time I was in the peer-counseling group, I became close

with three other women. The four of us had all experienced trauma
and were similarly trying to figure out spiritual paths in our lives.
We started exploring and developing different practices such as
meditation, which has increased my dialogue with my internal self
tenfold. The connection with my inner spirit has helped me take on
the stuff that happens in everyday life, which then makes me feel
more empowered to go further and further.

Without my connections with these women, I never would
have been able to build trust in myself or in others, nor to have a
healthy relationship with a man. I'm deeply emotional and deeply
interested in relationships. Expressing one's self and one's emotions to the fullest, at all points, isn't a practice regularly supported
by society. With my circle of women friends, I've gotten to express
and honor this emotional side of myself, and without this support I
wouldn't feel as grounded in who I am. The biggest thing my group
does for me is support me when I'm in those moments of doubt.
They always believe in me; they're 100 per cent, "You are going to
make it."

Of course I have my more confident days as well as my less
confident ones, but now the difference between the two is discern-
able. If I'm not feeling it, I can say no to sex. When fear or self-doubt
show up, I give myself space to figure it out and don't pretend to
be interested. I had to come to this on my own. I needed to find my
voice in my sexuality. In the past I've had a hard time talking about
things I wanted and things I didn't. Through practice—through
using my voice more—and through the internal work I've been
doing, being sexual has gotten easier. If there's any point where I
don't think I'll be able to share my voice, I will stop what's going on
and give myself time to meditate on it. Or, if we're having sex and

something comes out of someone's mouth like, "Ooo you're a bad girl," I'll be quick to say, "No, that is *not* how I get down." It took a while to reckon with that! I used to second-guess myself, thinking this is someone being playful with their sexuality—maybe I'm getting too heavy. I'd worry how would this man deal with that? I've gotten to a point where I don't give a fuck: this is who I am and where I'm at. Having confidence in being sexual makes me feel strong. I've also gotten a lot better at picking men with whom to be in partnership. This ability has been many years in the making.

At this writing I'm about to turn 33, so I've been thinking about whether or not I want to recommit to this no-intercourse goal for one more year. I haven't decided. There have been multiple times when I was being intimate and I thought, "Fuck it, let's do it." And for whatever reason, I didn't do it. Now that I'm close to the end of the year, I'm glad I haven't had sex. My sexuality used to be influenced externally by what the men in my relationships wanted, or by what society was projecting, or by what my friends were doing or saying they were doing, and now it's not. My sexuality is such a deeply intimate and personal experience that I don't care what other people are expecting.

If *I* can get to an empowered place to decide my sexuality, I believe it's possible for anyone.

I don't want people to think I've got everything figured out. I surely don't want people thinking to themselves, "I don't have it figured out, what's wrong with me?" I've had to go into my depths. I've had to face all my fear and humiliation around sexuality, and it was super hard at times. Experiencing sexual violence has impacted my whole life. It made me doubt myself and feel physically unsafe almost all the time. This has affected everything I've done; it has affected my health and even job opportunities. I don't use the terms "victim" or "survivor" now. I embrace all that has happened to me in my life because it's made me who I am, and I absolutely adore and respect who I am. That being said, I still think I would be an amazing person even if I hadn't gone through all that bullshit, so I'm not saying I'm glad it happened. It did happen and there's nothing I can do to change that. I no longer categorize anything in my life as positive or negative. I no longer evaluate or judge any aspect of my life or my history. It's all just a part of who I am.

Gradually, my process and transformation have opened up. I haven't reached Oz yet. I don't even know if Oz exists, but I'm going to keep moving toward it regardless of where others are headed. My sexuality is mine alone, and I will continuously determine its direction.

Tara Abrol, LMSW, lives in Brooklyn where she founded BIG Talks Workshops, proving that no talk is too BIG to have with young people. Tara leads young people in openhearted dialogue about the complex issues affecting their lives such as sexuality, relationships, race, and gender. Tara also provides training for parents, teachers, and youth workers on how to effectively engage young people in dialogue. She is the author of the forthcoming books Sex: It's Something to Talk About *and* Sex: It's Something to Talk About: Parents' Companion Guide.

THERE BUT…

SAIDHBH

I like to write. For me writing is a sort of therapy, getting what's inside out without the vulnerability of verbalizing my experiences for someone else's consumption and possible judgment. Recently, I've revisited some of my written musings from over the years. I'd written them all in the third person because even the act of writing just for me couldn't provide a safe enough space where I could claim my own story.

I decided that this time the narrative would be different, this time I would write in the first person.

At the time, I told no one. I didn't have the vocabulary to articulate what had happened to me. Coming from 1980s small-town Ireland, sex hadn't quite arrived in my home yet. Even *Dallas* was routinely turned off when it got too steamy!

For years I told no one. When, at 21, I did tell my mother, she pretended not to have heard and just continued watching TV. Her facial expression did not change. When I revisited this with her a few years later, again there was no reaction. This time I was prepared. This time I challenged her on it. Her first question was, "Who was it?" I think when you tell someone, they often want to know who was the monster behind the act, but as I found out after I told my best friend, people don't really want to know. They *think* they want to know, but then, once they realize that the person is just a regular guy, a guy they know and like, suddenly they don't want to know anymore. And this can leave you feeling that their knowledge of the rapist's identity somehow depletes your personhood as the victim of the rape. You can read the questions in their eyes: "What did she do?" "There's no way he'd do that." Or: "I told you he was no good for you." "What did you expect?"

So, by the time I'd spoken to my mother for the second time, I realized that as soon as she knew his identity, the rape would no longer be about me, but about her reaction to the news of who he was. It would have been about her, about him, about my naivety, my disobedience. It might even have been reframed as my fault.

She was annoyed when I didn't tell her. This, to her, was the most important part of my story. And so, the conversation became about anything other than the rape, anything but my need for reassurance, love, or even pity. Instead she was annoyed with me because I refused to identify him. And that was it. Conversation had. Case closed.

Twenty-five years on, I can understand her reaction better. She was powerless in the face of such exposition. She had failed in one of the central duties of her motherhood—she hadn't kept her child safe. So the only way she could deal with the news was to make it about something else. Sometimes we find it difficult to resist the urge to make another's story about us. This is human. And this is part of the wisdom I've etched from the trauma: sometimes I just have to sit, listen, show empathy and love, and let the story be the other's and not my reaction to it. Listening to stories of trauma can be traumatic, but it is our duty at the moment of the telling not to make it about us but to let the person we're listening to keep the story as theirs. For the telling and being heard is part of the process of healing, and taking someone else's story and internalizing it and coming up with solutions can leave them feeling unheard and further wounded.

At no stage did I think that the rape was something I should report to the police. How could I do that to him? To his family? To my family? No. This was best swept quickly and firmly back under the carpet where it belonged. So I swept it under the carpet and for years that's where it stayed.

I didn't look at it again until I was asked for the first time why it had taken me so long to come out as a lesbian. I'd never given it much thought and fell back on the old reliables: small town Ireland, two TV channels, dutifully religious in my youth. When I reflected on it, however, I realized that one reason was that when I first considered I might be lesbian, I had immediately banished the idea. I was afraid that *thinking* I might be lesbian was just a response to the rape, and I felt that such an "unauthentic lesbianism" would be disrespectful to both lesbianism and lesbians! Prior to the rape, I was only beginning to develop a consciousness about my body and my sexuality; the trauma of the rape left me confused about my sexuality—not in the narrow sense of sexual identity, but sexuality in its broadest sense. It left me with a distanced and fractured relationship with my body. As a result, it took me years of agonizing self-reflection and self-doubt before I definitively came out, safe in

the knowledge that my lesbianism wasn't a curious by-product of
being raped.

I passed out during the rape from the pain and from the fact
that his hand was firmly over my mouth constricting my breathing.
When I regained consciousness, he was tying a knot on a condom
and dropping it over the headboard. (The following morning I
looked; there were lots of condoms there.) I didn't know enough
at the time to be grateful that he had used a condom. He promptly
rolled over and went to sleep without saying a single word to me.

I was sore, humiliated, and utterly and totally confused. I had
never thought about having sex. I know that in today's world this
sounds ridiculous, but I hadn't. I loved children and wanted to have
them when I was older, and so my biggest fear that early winter's
morning was that I would not be able to have children. My overwhelming feeling was panic. I tormented myself with questions
such as: *Had I had sex? Could I have sex? Was I even capable of it? If I
couldn't have sex would that mean that I couldn't have children?* This last
dread consumed me and is the one I clung to and panicked about as
I lay there, smoking cigarette after cigarette. Was I broken? Defi-
cient? I'd have to work out whether I could have sex and if I could
have children. What was possible? Knowing this established itself as
the most pressing priority of my young life.

I've heard that when trauma first comes back, it comes in
images, not words. This made sense to me because the things
that were strongest for me in the wake of the rape were disjointed
images: The hole in the curtainless window; the stark winter tree
standing motionless outside, observing the scene; the smoke of my
cigarette furling as I lay in bed, waiting to get up, afraid to sleep; my
copy of *Lady Chatterley's Lover* on the floor, a book he'd borrowed

from me and would never return. A book I had bought to seem older and sophisticated, but had never read. Would never read. Thinking back to the book now, there's a certain, almost comical, irony to it.

After he fell asleep, I lay there for hours, waiting until I heard his sister go to the toilet, and then I got up. The rest of the morning is a bit of a blur, but I can remember leaving the house with his brother and his friends and heading for the road and the long, cold ordeal of hitching our lift back to Kerry. The four-hour journey took us an unprecedented 12 hours. He hadn't said one word to me the whole time I was in Galway.

And when he was in Kerry next, he called and was kind and thoughtful and apologetic about his girlfriend whom I'd met in Galway (who wasn't *really* his girlfriend... I'd "misunderstood"). And I agreed to meet him. He was lovely. He kissed me. He took me home. Lit candles. Put on Van Morrison's "Into the Mystic." And he slowly and carefully had sex with me. I just lay there, not moving, not making a sound. He finished. Tied a knot on the condom. Put it over the headboard of the bed. Turned over and fell asleep. This time he kissed me first. I lay there. Sore and confused, the first seeds of self-loathing beginning to take root. But happy that at least I could have sex without passing out. I didn't like sex, but at least I had the capacity and capability. I would be able to have children.

I continued to have sex with him on and off for about a decade. He had this weird hold over me. Each time I'd swear that this would be the last time I'd let myself fall for his charms. I was so thoroughly ashamed of myself. Even all these years later I still feel a sense of shame. I thought the only way that I could attract or hope to keep someone was to have sex with them, which resulted in self-loathing and a lot of shame and embarrassment over the years. I cringe to think that this is part of my past, part of who I am. The only positive thing to come of it was that, with time, I became more sexually confident. For a long time I didn't realize that it was possible, as a woman, to enjoy sex. And so I didn't even really try. Most men I had sex with were happy enough to just please themselves and pay absolutely no attention to me. Then, when I was 25, after a couple of beers, my friend Jason and I found ourselves in bed together, and I had enjoyable sex for the first time, marking a shift in my relationship with my body and my sexuality.

This encounter, a one-night-stand with a friend, awakened in me the knowledge that it was possible for me to enjoy sex. It wasn't just something I had to do to get guys to like me; it could be something that I could get pleasure from. I remember when he asked me what I liked, the question and its implication were so alien to me that I couldn't even begin to dream up an answer. So he took what seemed like the entire night to help me discover what it was that I enjoyed. I was beginning to realize that desiring certain things, even thinking about sex and what I might like, was something to be explored and celebrated and not to be banished in embarrassment. Interestingly, it was also around this time that I started to question my sexuality in terms of my lesbianism, as if my relationship with the act of having sex needed to begin to repair before I could even think of who I wanted to sleep with. And by the time I finally came out, my experience of and attitude toward sex had shifted significantly. Sex was no longer something that at best, didn't interest me, or was, at worst, something I had to endure. I began to learn about sex through my engagement with it as something I could enjoy and explore. It represented a space where I could negotiate my sexual identity, identify my sexual needs, and have them met.

When I think back to this period now, and think of the generous, kind, attentive lovers I had before I came out, I wonder whether it was important for me to experience enjoyable sex with men in order to develop a healthy relationship with my own sexuality. If I had only ever had functional, unenjoyable, and bad sex with men, and had only experienced enjoyable and good sex with women, would this have caused me to construct a dichotomous relationship between sex and gender in my mind that would be unhelpful in my dealing with the rape? Would such dichotomous construction have resulted in my conflating badness with men and goodness with women? Either way, I'm glad that I had enjoyable sex with men, and genuinely believe that this has played a part in my development into a sexually confident woman. I discovered and explored the continuum that is sexual satisfaction from the nuances of emotionally fulfilling sex to the raw thrill of sex for the sake of sex. Sex expanded to represent different things at different times; it became something that could meet different needs. It could be fun, enjoyed, savored.

I can't know what my relationship with my body and my sexuality would have been had I not been raped. What I do know, though, is that almost 30 years on, I feel secure and confident in my body and sexuality. The fracture that the rape caused in my relationship with my sexuality has healed and I'm happy with who I am, sexually speaking. So while I could never be happy that I was raped, it is part of me. It is deeply woven into my sexual history and sexual identity. I am thankful that it did not break me, for it could have. And, trite as it may sound, it made me stronger and is impli-cated in the very fabric of my strength.

Since starting to write about this, I have occasionally reflected on why I was drawn to do so to begin with, and why I found myself unable to just walk away when I was tired of it and no longer wanted to finish it. Part of my reason for persevering is my belief in the value of story. When we are unable to speak the unspeakable trauma of our own experience, it can help to read someone else's story in which we can identify ourselves. We can feel pity for and empathize with another person and in this way learn to feel pity and tenderness for ourselves. The space created when we listen to another woman's story can open up a space within us where words attach themselves to the trauma of our own experiences. In this way it is in the experiences of other women that we can find the words and strength for our own healing.

Saidhbh lives and works in Dublin.

One Woman, Many Names

Sally J. Laskey

I clearly remember the day when I *stopped* being the Rape Lady.

As an undergraduate, I was a rape prevention educator and part of the Athletes for Awareness program. I did presentations about consent, healthy relationships, and sexual assault in residence halls, fraternity houses, and locker rooms. I also volunteered at the campus rape crisis center. For three years of my life, my date book (remember those?) was full with crisis line shifts and workshop schedules. I liked the work so much that I ended up becoming a staff person at the rape crisis center and spent another six years talking about sexual assault and healthy sexuality. This is when folks started calling me the Rape Lady.

They meant it in a loving way, mostly, and I don't think they realized the visceral response in my body every time I heard those words. First, I really dislike the term lady. Second, as a survivor of sexual assault, having "Rape Lady!" shouted at me just about every day as casually as they would say "Pizza Guy!" seemed to both heighten and diminish my own experiences with sexual violence. There was a time when I thought this would always be my name.

I have flourished and mended my spirit in different ways and multiple times over the years. Some friends have called me a phoenix. Experiencing a sexual assault my first year of college broke my spirit, sense of self, and confidence. I had to fight to find myself again, and in doing so I found a different self. I became energized to help others. Working at a rape crisis center for almost ten years was the most important thing I have done, totally worth the pain and distress associated with being called the Rape Lady. I feel that I was able to help many individuals and the community as a whole. I saw true courage, immense growth, and more commitment to the cause than can be captured with words. While this all fed my passion for justice, my soul wasn't being fed.

We didn't know enough about vicarious trauma at that time to set up sufficient supports for staff and volunteers. I was surrounded by some of the best people on the planet and I was a really good advocate for others, but I felt like a cancer was growing inside me and it was getting stronger and stronger each day. I started to think of *myself* as the Rape Lady. I was becoming one-dimensional. I realized that I needed a little bit—or maybe a lot—of distance. So I moved 500 miles away to work with a national nonprofit to help build the support structures for preventing and ending sexual violence and left the Rape Lady behind.

I was at my new job for about two years when the local mechanic who worked on my car referred to me as "the Sex Lady that worked at the Sex Center." At first I started to correct him, and then I stopped. This became a celebrated moment in my life where someone understood that I was working *for* something and not just *against* something.

No more Rape Lady. I'm the Sex Lady.

I don't mind being called the Sex Lady—and yes, absolutely, I'm happy to go with you to pick out a vibrator, or to help you tell a three-year-old about when and where it's okay to tickle his own penis, or to field any other tricky questions from the young people in your life. Healthy sexuality is what I do.

My mother always said that I was born with an agenda and I have always had my sexuality on that agenda. I have always had a healthy sexual relationship with myself. I have sensed and been connected to my sexual energy as long as I can remember: It has only been other people who have tried to interfere with or interrupt this relationship. Whether it was the boy in high school who video-taped my boyfriend and me being intimate without our knowledge; the girlfriends who judged me for liking sex "too much"; or the college boyfriend who always saw me as a rape survivor first and a human being second, I was able to break through that distraction and negative noise by reminding myself that my sexuality is about me and not about my relationship to others. If I don't "dig" myself and build and celebrate my sexual health, then I won't be fulfilled.

That said, I have had and maintain amazing relationships that have helped me explore my sexuality in astonishing, positive ways. Before Eve Ensler penned the monologue about "Bob"—an ordinary guy who loved to look at vaginas—for her play *The Vagina Monologues*, I met my very own "Bob." My Bob wasn't ordinary in any way, shape, or form, though. He was extraordinary in that he loved vaginas even more than Eve's Bob. I think my Bob wished that he had been born with a vagina. My Bob also worked in the anti-sexual violence movement and I felt that we were vagina warriors and peacemakers. I spent over a decade in a committed relationship with my Bob, exploring my vagina in the most playful and passionate of ways, and we remain the closest of friends. I am grateful for all of the gifts and lessons we shared.

Sexual violence isn't about sex, but it can have a significant impact on our sexuality and sexual health. Being in a sexual relationship with an anti-sexual assault activist—someone who "gets it"—was powerful and empowering. Having the space and time to figure out what "healthy" looked and felt like was crucial to me.

If I choose to be in sexual relationships with people, that means we need to be able to talk to one another about our needs and desires. *The Survivor's Guide to Sex* by Staci Haines was such a powerful tool for me and many other sexual assault survivors I have met. I think that we need a book for activists about how to do sexuality self-care work.

As a survivor, I have been exposed to health risks that require me to think differently about healthy sexuality; however, I didn't always think about how my activism work brought additional risks. It is just like the emergency instructions on a plane. I must affix my own oxygen mask before I can assist others.

∴

The anti-sexual violence movement was developed by survivors, and is often the voice of survivors. As it has been professionalized, some survivor voices within and outside the movement have been silenced. I want to work to keep these lines of communication open so that our community can work on healing from within while we are helping to create healing spaces for others.

While I loved being in a relationship with a fellow activist, I have to say that my current relationship with a son of a preacher, English major, mechanic-by-day, musician-by-night, and all around creative creature has been transformative. We met seven years ago. He makes me laugh and he supports my activism work, and sex is just a nice bundle of fun, love, and connection, rather than the political act it once was. The personal is still political in every way, but I have created sacred space in my current relationship that is protected from the outside world. Plus, it helps that I don't have a crisis line beeper going off in the middle of having sex or making lasagna.

I get to work with extraordinary people from around the country and the globe, who are wise, kind, and fierce in the best way possible. These survivors and anti-sexual violence activists are my family and my community. I find joy in figuring things out with them and in how we inspire each other to do even better for survivors and ourselves. I feel strong in this work and every day my partner reminds me how strong I am in many other contexts. I love sharing our lives and creating a future together.

I have high expectations for myself; I can't help it, I'm the daughter of two teachers. Generally this works well for me, though I've had to take a step back as I enter menopause, or what I like to call puberty in reverse. My partner and I have agreed that we expect each other to take care of ourselves to the best of our ability and to ask each other for anything that we might need—and to understand that we might not always get it. I now work mostly on simply paying attention to my body, my needs, and my spirit and being kind to myself. My sexuality is mine, and it is constantly changing.

And I'm sure that to many, I will always be known as the Sex Lady.

Sally J. Laskey resides in Pennsylvania, but her heart remains in Maine where she grew up, though her mother routinely refers to her as her daughter "from away." She is a community psychologist and has worked as an anti-sexual violence activist all of her adult life.

FOUR OUT OF FIVE
GLEN

I've never felt like a victim; these "things" just happened. My age when they took place and my attitudes toward each different event and each different abuser—all four, well, five—are as varied as the offences themselves. The one constant throughout is that each offender was significantly older than I.

As a 15-year-old boy in a sexual relationship with an 18-year-old girl, I was well chuffed with myself for being the object of desire for a female three years my senior, but in the back of my head I wondered: *Why the hell would she want to have sex with a 15-year-old boy?* It seemed bizarre. When I turned 18, the thought of me being in a sexual relationship with a 15-year-old girl was unfathomable, incomprehensible, and fucking creepy. The crime is statutory rape. There's no grey area; the lines are pretty freakin' clearly defined. Yet, everybody was complicit in this: my mother, older sibling, schoolteachers, and friends. I've recently become a father and this experience has galvanized my thoughts on the matter: It is innately weird to want to have sex with a minor when you're an adult. I would not condone it in any way, shape, or form if any of my children were either the victims or the perpetrators.

My "experiences" I wear almost like badges of honor. I have always been happy to talk about them and have, for the most part, retold these stories with humor. To me, they are hilarious accounts of weird moments in my life and I am always surprised when people are horrified by what I am telling them. Basically, it's a story about a sexual predator dressed up as a good yarn. I'm recounting the story, I'm here, I'm good, they're fucking creepy, life's weird, 'ey? I feel like these events in my life are like chapters in an absurd self-help book. I even have the title and a couple of ideas for the book:

Your Guide to a Better Life

…When playing with an older boy and you suddenly (yep, that's how it happens, before you know what's hit you) find him behind you with your pants down and his penis in your bum and he says, "Now it's my turn," if you don't want to put your penis in his bottom, instead place your index finger between his butt cheeks and thrust your hips backwards and forwards. He'll be happy. You don't even have to go anywhere near the hole. Everyone's pants get pulled up. He'll go home and you'll never have to play with that kid again.

Or so I thought… at that point I still had no real understanding of what had happened beneath my mother's elevated bed where previously I had happily enjoyed recreating all of my favorite musically-inspired *Star Wars* moments, and had sung along to hundreds of rotations of Meat Loaf's *Bat Out of Hell.*

Sometime after my happy place was ruined, I found myself an overnight guest at this same boy's house. Maybe staying the night at his house was a prior arrangement that I felt I needed to honor. Maybe it was the same day. I don't know anymore. His bedroom was in a converted garage that he shared with his 20-year-old brother. I remember not being able to sleep at all that night, desperately waiting for first light so I could walk home. I was terrified. I don't know why, I don't know what of—all I remember is being scared, probably the most scared I have ever been in my entire life.

When I stopped playing with that kid, the fear passed. I did not feel any shame; something bad had happened to me, and similar to losing a game of football or doing poorly in an exam, I got over it and went about playing with kids who didn't want to fuck me in the bum. It's funny because it's true.

I have realized in my journey that I've used humor as a means to not only resolve any issues I may have had, but to take ownership of these events and make them into stories of resilience and quick thinking. My experience as the victim of sexual assault has taught me to be observational, cautious, and canny.

I feel I'm perceptive, especially when it comes to assessing dangerous or potentially dangerous situations. I can be wrong at times (Nobody bats 1000!), but often I'm spot on. Please, join me on a wee journey as we travel back to the mid 80s, to a group of 15-year-old boys...not bad boys, just naughty. Well one day, an actual real life "bad boy" turns up at school and joins their clique. Within the space

of two weeks, these boys are transformed from petty thieves stealing change out of unlocked cars into car thieves…

One Saturday night, full of grog, the boys set out to do what
they—okay, what we always did on a weekend night—find an
unlocked car and loot it for money, cassette tapes (remember the
decade), and even a pewter mug with the engraving *Happy Birthday!*
We love you Daddy! (I always felt a bit bad about that one). Stupidly, I
assume that the "bad boy" is looking for coins on the floor or trea-
sure under the seat, when in fact he's under the dash hotwiring the
car. Before I have time to think, he has started the car, yelled for us
to get in, and off we drive. Exhilaration is quickly overtaken by fear:
the fear of getting caught; the fear of having an accident. We were
all liquored up and felt a real fear of the riskiness of this situation. I
want to get out of the car—I am shit-scared. I also know that if I tell
them I want to get out of the car because I am scared, I won't be let
out. I need a plan and I need it quick.

"I need a piss!"

"What?"

"I really need a piss."

"Now?"

"Yes, now! I'm going to piss my pants."

The "bad boy" stops the car and I get out. "I'm going to walk
home," I say. My "mates" call me a bunch of names: *gutless, poofta,*
chicken… And rubber burning, they speed off down the street.

I step outside early the next morning, and the car we'd stolen has been abandoned/parked across the footpath at the top of my street, with its engine still running. A statement, I think, designed to intimidate/bully me. I'll be honest, it worked.

Anyway, I feel this event is one of those moments you can pinpoint where you make a choice that makes a significant impact on the rest of your life. How so, you ask? While I chose to leave the vehicle and go home, the car's remaining occupants spent the weekend stealing more cars. On Monday while I was at school, they broke into the house of a school chum because they knew his parents always had boxes of cigarettes in their house. What they didn't bank on was the mother coming home while they were in the house. The mother was bashed and they fled with the cigarettes.

So what has that trip down memory lane got to do with being sexually assaulted? Everything! You become aware. You become a better judge of character. You teach yourself to listen to that voice in your head and that feeling in your gut. You learn to improvise ways to handle the situation: I've burst into tears to avoid getting my head punched in by an older and exceedingly tougher guy than me. "Whatever is required," that's my motto (if I had a motto, that is).

That's bullshit. My motto would probably be something along the lines of: "Respect everyone and everything and don't be a cock-head."

I think my experiences have given me clarity. I am able to process information, see potential dangers, and take an appropriate course of action quickly.

Two of the sexual assaults were committed at roughly the same time period in my life (when I was eight and nine), by persons of each sex, in totally non-related incidents. With the male (11 or 12-years-old), I clearly remember not wanting to participate and not being aroused. With the female (also 11 or 12), I was an aroused, curious, and willing (albeit strongly persuaded), participant. My primary concern about participating in these activities with the older female was that I might impregnate her. I can't remember if sexual intercourse occurred. What I do remember is her insisting that we have sex, and every time I said that I didn't want to, she repeated that it was OK, and that she wouldn't get pregnant. It's fucking gross to remember.

Seriously, I'm fine about all of this "stuff." Yet, the predatory nature of assaults upon a younger and physically and emotionally weaker person angers me. What saddens me is that I don't feel that I am unique or special for having lived these experiences. In fact, for a number of reasons, I feel quite ordinary. Firstly, I feel that these assaults were tame compared to the violence that I know others have experienced. Secondly, I know sexual offence is disgustingly commonplace. I have found ways to put these events behind me, and while I can speak openly and freely about them (mostly), there are lots of people who cannot, and I am overwhelmed with empathy for them. It breaks my heart.

Each time I was a victim of a sexual assault, I was in my own home or in the care of someone my mother had left me with. I don't blame her. My mother loves me deeply and would probably be mortified if I told her in any detail about what has happened to me. She was and still is a good mother. Yet everything that happened to me happened on her watch.

As a new parent myself, I have the mindset that you can't be too careful. Take for example, the man in the red suit. I've been a shopping center Santa Claus for the last six years. Now, *I* know I'm not a pervert, but how does anyone who puts his or her child on my knee know I'm not a pervert? They don't. They can't. Your kids don't have to sit on Santa's knee! Rather, suggest that they stand beside him or sit next to him. Keeping the kids off Santa's lap is win-win: If Santa *is* a pervert, you've kept them off his lap. If Santa is a great guy, then keeping them off his lap is also a win. "How is that a win?" I hear you ask. Consider this: The Santa suit is hot, really freakin' hot! And children are like tiny little furnaces. Also, Santa doesn't think it's cute when children are pulling at his beard, or kicking him in the nuts. Win-win.

I am extremely comfortable being the protective parent. Others can judge me harshly and say that I am "shadowing" my three-year-old, but experience has taught me a thing or two. The drawback to being proactive, trying to foresee all possible negative outcomes to every situation, and taking steps to avoid trouble, is that I look like an overprotective idiot. (See! This is what happens. Self-doubt. Maybe I am an overprotective crackpot. Maybe my danger-sensing powers ain't what I think they are. Maybe one day, I'll allow myself to follow the lead from others and loosen my protective and cautious grip on my children. Methinks not. I will remain cautious and never know, rather than choosing to ignore my gut and regret it.) I *am* that well-meaning father that everyone wishes would just fuck off, and I wear this title with immense pride. My children will not find themselves in the same awkward situations that I experienced. Granted, they may find themselves in other equally awkward experiences that I cannot foresee or do anything about. But, with God/Allah/You as my witness, I will be their Shepherd where I had none.

Or so I thought…

I took my family (girlfriend and two kids) to visit my father for his birthday. Dad had invited us out for breakfast, and at the café I was doing my usual "shadowing the son" routine, so I missed a poignant conversation. My girlfriend told me on the drive back home that Dad's significant other, whom the teen-aged me used to call The Ginger Ninja, commented she thought it was hilarious that I am exactly the same way with my son (overprotective, paranoid, and shadowing) as my father was with me when I was a wee one. Normally I wouldn't have given that remark a second thought, but writing and remembering for this project got me thinking:

I know that my father had a challenging upbringing, and I wonder if his reasons for shadowing me mirror my reasons for shadowing my son?

For all of my joking and the façade of being at peace with what has happened to me, there is one sequence of events with one particular offender that is the exception. (What's a rule without an exception?) I have not shared this story with anyone and won't here, but the older I get, the angrier, more resentful, and embarrassed I become. Not embarrassed by the event itself, but by the stigma attached to such a thing. So, for those who have kept silent, I get it. I understand why you can have insecurities and harbor feelings of anger and resentment, and how the whole thing can make you feel so dirty and ashamed that you dare not tell a soul. I toy with the idea of talking to someone about it because I feel that I'm at that point in my life where I would be okay if I did talk about it. Also, I want to expose the predator for who they are and what they did.

And I have no idea how that hand, when laid down, will play out. Is it even worth going down that path? Maybe it is, if only to give those closest to me insight into why I have reservations about this individual.

I understand how these events can fuck with how you feel about yourself. There are a lot of dickheads in the world. I had the misfortune of crossing paths with a few of them. I was in the wrong place at the wrong time. I didn't do anything to deserve it or to provoke it. In time, I will share this story with someone I trust deeply, most probably my girlfriend and mother of my children, and when I do, I am confident that I'll spin it into a yarn for the ages.

Glen is a musician and an actor, but don't hold that against him. He sings in a band, but he is not a vain, self-absorbed wanker. His secret power is that he is un-offendable. He is the proud father of two grouse kids with his bloody fantastic lady friend.

BODY, HEART, DESIRE

Trúc Anh Kiều

When I was a child, my body was my playground, my girlhood was a gem that I held in my hand with a gentleness free of judgment or fear. I can still remember the delight and awe I experienced when I gave myself orgasms as a child. Such pleasure was free, consensual, and wholly mine.

Obviously, it felt good to touch myself. I did it often, so much so that my older brother would yell, "Ew! Don't touch me! Your hand smells like butt!" I learned to wash my hands. And yet, before self-conscious thoughts overtook, before I owned a mirror, before the shame and silence settled in, I felt complete. My sense of self was seamless: soul and body, need and want, me. I didn't know then that those years of fearless exploration, discovery of my sexual self, and feeling of completeness would become things that I would desperately yearn to return to as an adult.

This feeling of completeness was lost to me (but not destroyed or tainted or broken) when an older man, a friend of my parents, started touching me without my consent. The routine messages I received as a child about modesty and chastity—"Close your legs!" "Sit like a girl!" "Be modest!"—helped to build a wall of silence that protected him. I kept his secret as I endured years of unwanted touching. Somehow along the way, I lost the knowledge of how to be complete.

When I arrived at college I mimicked others to fit in, so I hooked up with random partners. My sexual encounters were ephemeral things, and I would joke to my friends that I was a one-hit wonder. I chased after sexual experiences that I wanted, but still, hooking up felt transactional and mindless. I was open, yet closed.

My heart existed separate from my body. Sometimes they spoke, but they were like two people in a conversation who didn't know how to listen. They interrupted each other, cut each other off, and had nothing in common. They did not understand each other, and it became impossible to satisfy either of them. Sex and intimacy became monsters in my life.

One day, after a steady string of disappointing sexual encounters that were devoid of any pleasure, I realized that I had absolutely no fucking idea what it was like to feel sexual desire for someone. I looked at my friends who were on such different (and positive!) sexual journeys from mine. How would it feel, I wondered, if I could be like them? Like normal, I thought. I came to the conclusion that I was fucked up.

Enough was enough. I wanted to want. I wanted my heart and body to reconnect. I needed to heal. I needed connection. I wanted to experience sex and actually feel something.

Resolute in trying a new direction, I took on the task of solving or "fixing" myself: I was the one choosing these sexual partners. I was the one who didn't know how to be in healthy relationships. I was the one who didn't understand how to integrate sex and intimacy. If I was the problem, if I was creating a monster out of myself, then I could solve it. "It" being me.

I couldn't have been more wrong.

I fell in love for the first time when I was 22 years old and it felt like a million sunbeams lighting up my universe. When I thought about him, I felt butterflies in my stomach—I had only read about this in novels or imagined in movies. When we spent time together, we talked. He wanted to hear my thoughts and opinions, and we laughed all the time.

When we kissed, I felt like my cells were all reverberating, humming with happiness.

When I told my partner about my childhood, he listened. I have never felt so heard, so seen, and safe. (Although "safe" doesn't seem to be the most accurate word to describe the feeling, it'll have to do.)

I read that humans heal from hurts, betrayals, and trauma in layers. Healing, in other words, doesn't happen all at once. While I was filled with joy experiencing this new love, the ugliness of my own pain caught me off-guard. One night, we were making love for a long time when my partner suddenly stopped and said, "I just want to hold you."

Baffled, I grappled with my feelings of rejection.

"Do you not…want me?" I asked.

My words hung in the air, and I started to feel self-conscious lying naked beside him. He made a sound of surprise that quelled my doubt, and he wrapped his arms around me in a big hug.

In that moment, I realized I am still learning to recognize what love looks like. That moment illuminated an assumption I had—that sex was the pinnacle of love, that my worth was tied to how well I could please my partner. I was happy to be wrong.

bell hooks wrote, "When we love we can let our hearts speak." That night, my body and my heart reached for one another. Without the mutual respect my partner and I had for each other I wouldn't have had the courage to voice that question, or had the chance to shed yet another layer of hurt.

Now, I know that love can be a hug. I know that love can be listening to one another. And I know that sex can be transformative and healing in many ways. I also know that I can love and affirm myself, no partner needed. Now that I know these things, I see myself with an infinite capacity to love myself and to love others.

There is still distance between my body and my heart, but fear no longer blocks my path to healing. I am starting to feel complete.

Trúc Anh Kiều is a first-generation Vietnamese-American living in Minneapolis. She earned a Bachelor's Degree in Sociology/Anthropology and Women & Gender Studies from Carleton College in 2014. This is her first published work.

BECAUSE I LOVE HARD

TOLD BY NEFER BOVEA
COMPOSED BY CATHY PLOURDE

My partner got me a massage for Christmas. I said, "What part of 'I don't like massages' do you not understand?"

He said, "I know you don't like massage, but this is different. It's a hot stone massage, and I think it can help address the hesitancy you have about being touched... um, Merry Christmas, sweetie?"

He's right. I want to work on touch. I give my daughter soothing massages all the time, whispering to her, "Hey, doesn't this feel good?" so she can learn to appreciate touch.

I can say, for my short time being a mom, you have to give so much and that can be depleting. Sometimes it's enough just getting through the day, and it's important to think about how I replenish myself and make sure I'm OK in order to be able to nurture the ones I love. This is an ongoing theme in my life. Internally, I can be overly harsh with self-talk, and I have to undo that: it's about being kind to myself, thinking about the fun in living life, and even the fun in setting expectations. My expectations right now include committing to being in integrity with myself and others, to fully loving myself, to trying my best, to forgiving my mistakes, and to remembering that it is a process. My partner's gift of a massage promotes taking care of myself.

Motherhood for me is eye opening, and everything is exposed and messy. My daughter is turning one next month. I'm looking forward to that. She's growing, reaching developmental milestones, and I have so much love for her. I've liked watching her feel out how she wants to relate to me. I don't want to smother her. I want her to know she can deal with whomever she wants to deal with; she doesn't have to bend to anybody's rules on how she should be in this world. And teaching this to her changes the cycle of what children, particularly girls, are given as messages.

My relationship with my own mother has been tough at times. I've had a lot of anger, especially with how the trauma I experienced was dealt with, and how my sexuality was hindered as a result. But I also have compassion, because when my mother grew up, sexuality was a big void for her as well. Sex was not talked about with her, and so it was not talked about with me, either. As I get older I have a better understanding of her love for me. Our love continues to blossom in our mother/daughter bond, but for a time there was so much secrecy, shame, and silence between my mother and me. I do not want to create that for my daughter and me. This silence ends here. It's not that I want to share detailed information about my trauma experience, but I want my daughter to be comfortable about her sexuality and her body.

I was subjected to sexual abuse from age 5 to about 11. I didn't know what to do. Around age 11 or 12 I decided to speak up about it, and then I got judged. Heavily judged. A social worker made a report, and there was an investigation, and it went nowhere. Ties to the family friend ended but the damage was done. As a result my experience was filed away as, "This never happened, we're not talking about it." I was socialized that as a girl you sit with hands folded, you listen, you do what you're told, and you're not a rabble-rouser. I grew up Catholic and that social catechism is embedded in me, too.

Those messages scarred me. I think this is why I continue to work on speaking up.

Blame and heaviness shrouded me for a long time. I'm still uncovering and peeling off those layers of hurt. I've built courage to use my voice and share my opinion, even if I think what I have to say is silly, even if I'm afraid it won't make sense. Right now, I'm over and done with the shame. I'm done shouldering even the suggestion that it was my fault. It's not my fault, even though I was told I should've known better, that if I hadn't done *this* then *that* wouldn't have happened. No. I'm over that.

There was a turning point for me when I was 21. I was distraught and my close friend, who was like a sister to me, was also going through a hard time. We decided to take a three-month seminar involving weekly meditation and learning about tools of empowerment. The course met every Saturday, and we worked to understand mindfulness and staying in the present. The program gave me insight into how I wanted to live my life and how to not live in my past so much. Those three months rebooted my life.

It helps to do a lot of talking with like-minded people, and with people who recognize what you are going through. I barely graduated from college. I worked in social services for a time, but I never felt that was enough. Ten years later I went back to school for a Master's degree and developed a passion for higher education. I now work as an advisor in a community college because I understand how difficult it can be for those who are on the outskirts or who don't have a strong sense of self to navigate the college world. I love to support students' academic success because somebody believed in me when I needed it, and helped me to grasp where I fit in, and believed that I have value. Going back to graduate school was a risk—it made me vulnerable—and because I took the risk, I have learned more about *how* I matter. I still struggle with success and wonder if I belong, but I've found my way through different spiritual teachings and philosophies and I can now say, *I belong here. I did succeed.*

Prior to the relationship I'm in now, I felt as though I was broken. I wasn't able to handle relationships; anything that triggered a feeling of victimhood would turn into a fight, because I wasn't ready to talk about what happened when I was a child. I didn't know how to talk through my feelings. Being so entrenched in the hurt, I didn't have the tools to express myself in a way that wasn't going to damage the relationship. I would just pretend everything was fine and deflect away from what was really going on with me. I've gotten better at trusting that issues can come up and I don't need to hide or shy away. I can be angry and it's OK; I can be sad and it's OK.

In my 20s, I had a partnership that lasted for about 10 years. I appreciate that it provided some important life lessons I'd need for my 30s; on the other hand, aspects of it hindered my growth emotionally, and I have had a lot of anger about how long it was before I realized that relationship wasn't leading anywhere. Afterwards, I didn't date much but there were three or four tentative years of

exploring the dating world without being in a committed relationship. For a long time the burning question in the back of my mind
was, "When will they find out? Will I get triggered, and then have to
talk about it?" I feared that the person I was with would leave me.
As prevalent as sexual trauma is, abuse and sexuality are still taboo
topics. That's changing with social reform, policy, and even by dis-
cussions around the kitchen table, yet I feel it's going to be a while
for change to manifest for the masses that need it.

There are people I'm connected to on social media who have
experienced the same or similar trauma to mine. I know, because we
had the same abuser. I'm tempted to express support or ask if they
would want to talk about it, but I don't because it's not right for me
to put that on another person. I wish there was a space to talk about
it, to see how they were affected or how they worked through it, or
even if they admit any abuse occurred. It would be nice to be honest
and say, "Yes, we were young, and this happened, and how are you
doing now?"

In the past five years I have taken more ownership in reclaiming my sexuality. I feel more confident in my body and how I see
myself in the scheme of intimacy and pleasure, instead of feeling
that I was a mere service provider, very outside of me, a source of
pleasure for someone else. With my partner, my trauma history
came up organically. Because of the work I had done, I was able
to say, *Yes, that happened, and this is where I'm at.* He's been my gift
from the universe and he has helped me to find unconditional love
for myself. He is so compassionate and gentle and loving. His touch
can be warm and soothing; it expresses intimacy in ways that feel
good for me at times. And yet, what feels good and empowering can
sometimes trigger feelings I can't describe, feelings that undermine

the good and make me feel that I am doing something wrong. But now I know what this stems from: It's feeling vulnerable and the need for control. I've done a lot of work to improve how I deal with these feelings.

You have to do the work. Someone asked me, "What is that *work*? I don't know what the *work* is." It's difficult to say. You have to look at yourself critically, surround yourself with love, and find something that resonates with you. Labor and birth played an important role in my spiritual healing. I took a workshop on the chakras and sexual trauma, and while I was pregnant I did a lot of work on the second chakra, where I held my trauma. Birthing a child can clear this site for a fresh start. Instead, things were tough, both before and after the birth. I lost my job when I was three months pregnant and found myself trying to hide my belly on interviews. We had wanted a natural birth; however, after 39 hours of labor I had to have an epidural and a C-section, which resulted in an infection requiring hospitalization for two weeks. I had to take a close look at what I thought of the birth and how it triggered and compounded the old trauma, the feelings of pain, discomfort, and not being well. Over time I've found the birth of my child and my love for her has connected me more deeply to my healing.

I think it all goes back to love—and then comes the smarts, and then comes the compassion, and everything else follows. It all begins out of love for oneself. Unconditional love from my partner and from my friends has helped. Continuing to speak up and using my voice to share what feels good for me helps. Going to therapy and doing chakra work to release shame and to face my shadow side has allowed me to love and transform those hidden parts of me that I don't want to see.

While I did take time to create a concrete plan of action that had results, this is also a process. It's not, "Oh, I just healed—everything is great now." I feel guilt at times. I feel victimhood sometimes. But it doesn't overpower me the way it used to. I feel much more comfortable thinking and talking about the abuse, as opposed to hiding it. It took 10 or 15 years to get a start on recovery, and when I finally did, I surrounded myself with people who support me and challenge me on the journey to better understand myself and to fully enjoy my sexuality.

I like the way that my partner and I began exploring our sexuality together. I can be very modest in my dress and used to feel that if I *could* cover up everything all the time, I would. He helped me to build my confidence. There's beauty in the female body that's undeniable, and actually I love being naked; I love going around the house naked and feeling good in my body. I go to sleep in my underwear and when my daughter wakes me up, she sees me and touches me and explores my body. I want her to see that you don't have to cover up. I had a lot of body shaming in my life; reclaiming my body, and bringing that into my intimate relationship and into how I relate to my daughter and to the world has been a struggle. But it's a beautiful struggle. I like where I'm at right now.

As a child I had a lot of pressure to be perfect all the time. It was never *said* I had to be perfect. It was an unspoken expectation from my family and school and I internalized it early on. As a girl, I looked outside of myself for approval. I think I did that, in part, due to the trauma that I experienced. For me, at the forefront of partnership and motherhood is considering how to shape my daughter's experience of how she grows into her sexuality, and that means dealing with my own and others' expectations of having to do it all, and of getting everything right.

Because I've become more confident and self-assured, more self-aware and honest with my feelings, I'm more at ease being myself and having fun with reveling in the important relationships in my life, without worrying about safety or expectations. I'm happy that I'm flourishing—and happy to discover how much fun and joy there is in being able to put trust in people, in my partner and in my friends. When trust issues do come up, I look at what I am doing to create those walls, and then I look for ways to take the walls down, bit by bit. I'm able to talk about my healing process without feeling judgment. I'm loyal and committed to these people, and I love that my trust and love are received and reciprocated. Because I love hard.

Expressing your sexuality is a part of the human experience. We are sexual beings, period. Point-blank. The way we receive messages about sexuality can help us be confident, honest, and positive. In all the pictures of me as a young child, I'm posed with my hand on my hip smiling a really big smile; and now, every single time I'm having my picture taken, I still go to that pose. I like the fun I can have expressing my sexuality. It doesn't need to be shameful or feel dirty. It's an expression of who I am, on a continuum, a part of me and it doesn't need to be hidden.

Wrong was done to me but doesn't define who I am. I didn't have any power at that moment; however, I have power now, and in owning that power is happiness in knowing that I've come a long way. It's an unfortunate reality, but it didn't break me. I don't need approval or reassurance from others—it can come from me. People who have survived sexual trauma are often drawn to the helping professions, perhaps as archetypes of the "wounded healer," able to offer help to others in the healing process because of their own experience. That's been true for me, as I think about where I am and what my purpose is in this lifetime, and how I can contribute to minimize the wrongdoing of the world.

I do it for myself, and for my daughter. She's a part of the bigger picture.

Nefer Bovea is an academic advisor and has spent the last 15 years working with young people and their families from underrepresented communities in New York City. She resides with her partner and daughter in Brooklyn, New York.

My 24-Carat Self

Jordan Masciangelo

My feet ache, warm and swollen in my hiking boots. My whole body itches something fierce. A thick film of sweat and dirt slicks my face and arms as I trudge through the mud and undergrowth. It's not raining, but everything is wet and sloppy.

"They don't call it a rainforest for nothing," Eber tells me in his charming Spanish accent. A half-cocked grin of sarcasm breaks out on his face.

A freelance jungle guide, Eber knows these trails inside and out. He's walked them, lived them, and raised a family among them. He grew up on the outskirts of Rurrenabaque, a tiny town on the Beni River that acts as the Bolivian entrance to the Amazon. He is the jungle's Superman and I would have perished without his guidance and knowledge over the days we spent together.

He tells me to move quietly.

The sounds and songs of the rainforest charge at me from all directions, but there is also a strange silence. I am suddenly aware that I am insignificant among the vast tangle of trees and vines. For most of three decades, I had only fantasized about getting *out there,* traveling and experiencing life. *I put myself here.* I deliberately threw myself into what many would consider miserable and dangerous. With the clothes on my back and a small pack of provisions, I set off into the Bolivian Amazon to discover what I'm made of, to find the original me—what I call my 24-carat self.

Eber presses his index finger to his lips and points up toward the forest canopy. We've been tracking an elusive troop of capuchin monkeys for two hours and we've finally caught up to them. The incessant buzzing of a large jungle insect quiets as I come to a stop on the trail. This monstrous fly has been following and circling my head for so long now that she has synced her movement up with mine. At first, she was an itch I couldn't scratch. I ducked and swatted and cursed at her. While I was trying to be present and peaceful and experience the wild of the jungle, it seemed her sole purpose was to drive me absolutely mad. As the hours ran on and miles passed under my feet, she never once bit me and I began to realize her strategy; she's using me as her shield. Her protector. As long as she stays with me, anything coming after her will have to go through me first.

When I stop, she rests on my head. I can feel her six (or eight?) little legs tickling my skin. As soon as I take a step, she resumes her noisy salsa around my body. She moves fast and with purpose and she never wavers.

Maybe it was the heat, or the eight hours of hiking, maybe it was the solitude, or a combination of it all; I began to relate to that annoying jungle fly. I had been in that position many times in my life, vulnerable and alone in the big bad world, and much like her,

I was persistent and never gave up. That little (make that *massive;* nothing in the Amazon is little!) insect helped me crystallize what I have known all along: I am a fighter.

This jungle trek wasn't the first adventure I'd undertaken to gain perspective and reclaim the life that was skillfully stolen from me as a child, nor would it be the last. I was a survivor of childhood sexual abuse. I say "was" and I use the term "survivor" loosely because I don't think of myself as a survivor anymore. Survival was a stage in my recovery process, a grueling and sticky stage that can prove seductive and hard to leave—a lesson I wouldn't learn until seven years of therapy and adventures through nine countries were behind me.

The world is a scary place. We all know this. Most parents shield, protect, and try to prepare us for it. It's their job. Sometimes their efforts succeed and a lot of the time they don't, and that's OK. We figure it out on our own. My parents never sat me down to warn me to be careful around the ones I love, that they could have nefarious intentions. Why would they? People don't want to think about this happening.

But it does happen.

Trauma exhausts you and wears you down. Sexual trauma not only bends your mind, it warps it. It's a slow-acting poison. It disconnects you, twisting and reshaping your reality. It seeps into every facet of your being and slowly eats away at your body and mind until you are nothing more than a shell of what you once were. Nothing is safe from its grasp. The trauma takes over your life and you are its shadow, the person you were before only a vague memory.

I *do* recall those early years, the years that preceded the mess I was soon to become. I was born a happy child into a happy family, a chubby Italian boy surrounded by four brothers and sisters and loving parents. Life was simple and I was carefree. All that mattered was playing on my Nona's farm and raiding the chicken coop for eggs. My OshKosh overalls were always filthy because of my zeal to be outside, where I was mesmerized by nature and animals and the science of the world. "You were a funny kid. Your first word wasn't *mama* or *dada*, hon, it was *book*," my mother told me recently. On one birthday, my mother gave me a university-level textbook on human anatomy. It was fascinating. I didn't know what all the words meant but I remember staring at the images and marveling at how everything is connected, how the soles of your feet are so closely connected to the small of your back. I was an extrovert and a bookworm, somewhat of an oddball, and I relished my bubbly, off-kilter nature. Life was exactly how it should be. I was young and happy. I was innocent. I was pure.

All that light, all that exploration and discovery, ground to a life-changing halt when I was eight years old. The effects of divorce are worse for some than others, and for me, it was a hell that again, my parents hadn't prepared me for. My tiny happy life-bubble burst with such a sudden force it knocked the breath right out of me. It ripped my family apart so instantly and unforgivingly that none of us fully recovered. My siblings and I were caught in the fighting and the chaos. I felt like a pawn as we traveled back and forth between households. I didn't know whom I could trust so I withdrew and chose nobody. The natural joy that I used to find so easily, faded.

Turmoil molded me into a perfect target.

A family friend moved into my father's house and quickly became everything to me: a man I grew to trust, to love and confide in, a man that I could look up to as a father figure and as a best friend. He was going to save me, be the sun that burned through the storm clouds that had engulfed my world. I latched onto him and held tight. I bought his trick, hook, line, and sinker, and he betrayed me. He determined that his sexual pleasure could come at the expense of my growth and wellbeing as a young boy. He molested me.

Chronic sexual abuse went on for years and years right under my father's nose, and I grew further and further away from my 24-carat self.

Frankly, after the initial shock of the abuse, I got used to it. He repeatedly assured me that what was happening was OK, that we had a special relationship, a secret romance. I believed him. It was clear that all I had to do was submit to his sexual desires and he would *be* there for me. I so desperately needed someone that I was willing to pay the price: I wouldn't tell a soul. It didn't help that my mother remarried and my family and I were locked in as victims at the hands of my abusive step-dad. I developed an impenetrable shell and hid. My body matured but my mind stayed trapped in the trauma.

With nowhere to go, I left home, determined to conjure up an existence beyond what I had known. I wasn't a sorcerer and I had no spells or potions to escape the past. I was just a sixteen-year-old boy who knew how to hide and had only my wits to keep me alive. I *really* was alone now, figuratively and literally, and the emptiness consumed me.

They say you can't run from your past, but I tried. I ran from it, and I ran fast. I barely had time to adjust to my new surroundings in a new city before trauma's sharp talons found me and retightened their grip. My days soon filled with highs and lows and blades and blood. I fed the beast with drugs and self-harm, until that no longer sufficed to satiate its ever increasing appetite. I had to find something else. The unfortunate solution fell right into my lap.

I was wearing all black that night. Black jeans and black hoodie, characteristic of the monochromatic palette I had adopted to help maintain invisibility and anonymity in the world. It was important to be as non-descript as possible to help elude any law enforcement or authoritative presence. With my hood up and over my face like a Jedi knight, I sat tracing my finger over the lines in the cracked sidewalk and wracked my brain for how to gratify the monster inside me. A small black sports car pulled over and came to a stop no more than ten feet away from me. Head down, but curious, I raised my eyes from under my hood to see the tinted passenger side window slowly scroll down.

"Hey kid," a barely audible voice said from the darkness of the car's interior. At first I assumed the voice was referring to somebody else.

"Kid, come here a second," the voice whispered more loudly.

I raised my head a little higher and tried to see through the window, but my angle from the ground wouldn't allow it. The car idled. I waited for something to happen. Nothing did. I guessed it was my move. So with the thought that I had nothing to lose and maybe this voice would be what I was waiting for, I stood up.

"Me?"

"Yeah, you," the voice said.

I cautiously looked around. I stood up straight so as to not appear weak or vulnerable, and with feigned confidence I stepped up to the car and peered in the window. Inside sat a middle-aged man looking straight ahead, avoiding eye contact with me. He wore thick-framed glasses and had a noticeable bald spot, handsome in a way, but weathered-looking.

"You OK? Get in." He waved his hand gesturing for me to get in the car.

You would think at this point I would've walked away from this potentially dangerous situation, but my mind was clouded from the lifestyle I was living and the crushing pressure to feed the misery inside me. I opened the door and slid inside. I remember thinking I *should* be scared, but I wasn't. Fear couldn't stand in my way; the worst had already happened.

The specifics aren't necessary. The man offered me money in exchange for sex: I accepted. That night ushered in what I thought was sexual freedom. *I* was taking charge and making the decisions when it came to sex this time. I could use what I knew best and profit from it. Hustling made me feel powerful at first, something I hadn't felt since the abuse. As badly as I was treated by a lot of the johns, that flash of control and the desire to be wanted kept me going back. This worked.

I was wrong.

I took strange comfort in allowing myself to be abused and sexually mistreated over and over again. Like a familiar childhood blanket, I was used to its smell, its warmth. Once I got ahold of it again, I didn't want to let go. I felt that this was where I belonged, at the bottom of the barrel. I accepted it.

At that point in my life, I had no sexual identity whatsoever. I never concerned myself with the idea of being gay or straight or anything in between. All I knew was what I had been taught: Sex was secretive; I was good at it; and, I could use it to get what I wanted. So that's what I did with no regard to what I was doing to myself.

The sexual trauma piled up, layer upon layer, further skewing my view of sex and its place in the world and my life. There was no pretense of intimacy or pleasure. On one hand it seemed so easy and comfortable, and on the other hand I felt I had morphed into a hideous monster who would always be judged and reduced to being good for one thing only: a one-trick pony, as it were. The world was chock full of cruel and hateful people who couldn't wait to use me and rip me apart. I just wanted it all to end, but something in me, some puny flicker of light, wouldn't let me call it quits. I had fight in me yet.

It was hard to escape.

∴

One month before I walked with my guide, Eber, into the depths of the Amazon, I arrived in Panama City via an excruciatingly arduous and complicated bus ride from San Jose, Costa Rica. The nineteen-hour ordeal didn't bode well for my confidence in what I was getting myself into. I was the only non-local en route, and I hadn't heard or spoken a word of English the entire way. Upon arrival, I walked an unknown number of miles, with my pack in tow, to the hostel in Casco Viejo. As I walked up the winding stairs to my shared bunk on the top floor of the rickety old building, hordes of young adults flooded down, raging and laughing. The air was thick with sexual vibrations. It was as if I had walked into a Latin American frat house, with people standing in every hallway, chatting and telling stories, each trying to one-up the other. I was at least five years older than most. I plopped my pack down on my bed and pulled the scratchy blue privacy curtain across. The familiar feeling of panic and loneliness crept up on me like a thick fog as I sat there staring at the wall. I began to think that this solo traveling shtick was a mistake. I pulled out my smartphone and pinged Marc, my husband. I needed to hear his voice.

That voice has always had an effect on me. His goofy tone and the way he calls me "bear" immediately extinguish my self-doubt. It was like this from day one with Marc. We had met on a date, a date that I had zero faith in and nearly blew off because I was feeling sorry for myself. A date that turned into an inexplicable romance between two men simply meant to be with each other.

My phone pinged back and I stepped out onto the balcony to call Marc. The night air was hot and still, and I could hear the buzz of the parties from within the hostel. Instantly my husband's voice vanquished the feelings of panic and isolation. I stared out over the crumbly old buildings and the dim lights of the oldest part of Panama City as he asked me how the bus ride was. I didn't tell him about the feelings of doubt I was experiencing moments before because I didn't have to. They were gone.

"Are you having fun? I miss you tons," he said.

He wanted me to do this; he had pushed for me to do this, and then supported me the whole way through. *I could do this.*

Earlier that year, we had travelled Peru together. We hiked the Andes, sailed Lake Titicaca, and climbed the incredible Machu Picchu. Standing at the highest point of that ancient city, so delicately resting on the top of a mountain in the Peruvian jungle, I realized that this was for real. Getting out there, seeing the world, wasn't a dream or fantasy anymore. Hand in hand, we took in the epic vista and the deep beauty around us, and the appreciation I felt for that place and that moment was astounding. I was where I should be, marveling at this planet with a man I so dearly loved. We neared the final days of our trip, and we were walking the streets of Puno, looking for a *café con leche* to enjoy in the morning breeze. We were discussing how incredible the trip had been, how much I had fallen in love with Latin America and travelling in general.

We had spent three weeks in China only a few months prior. Marc had a thought:

"Why don't you come back?" he said. "Alone."

I looked at him.

"Seriously?"

I had fantasized about solo backpacking a foreign land since I was young, and I never had the means or the gumption to do it. He knew this, of course.

"We'll plan it." He smiled. "Quit your job, I'll support you, and you can come back here to South America for your thirtieth birthday. Pick a bunch of countries, take a few months to see and do what you want, and when you get home, we'll start over. Together."

I was ecstatic and scared all at the same time. Marc knew, more so than I did, that a solo adventure would not only make one of my dreams come true, it could also be a way for me to purge the past two decades of shit, and herald in a new beginning with a fresh perspective. He was willing to support me. He knew that my need, my desire to do this was not a reflection of anything to do with him or our relationship as it stood. His offer was selfless and nurturing, and although he was basically sending me off for months alone, I had never felt so loved and so connected in all my life.

Connection had always been a tough one for me, especially as the only significant connection I had felt in the past 15 years was with my abuser—a connection that had been severed with a dull knife. With that betrayal, I walled up my heart, and I would hold it captive for years, safely stashed where nobody could find it, nobody could touch it. No, no one would get that close again.

I had learned to fake connection as a teen on the streets, to *act* like I loved so as to not reveal the secrets I had cleverly buried inside. The act was invaluable when it came to sex, when it came to hustling, and when it came to making people believe that they knew me. The more a john felt as though we had a connection beyond just the sex, the more I'd get in return: more money, better drugs, nicer hotels. I kept them coming back. I thought I was being powerful, savvy. I deserved an Academy Award.

After years of therapy and recovery, my heart still remained closed off. The only real difference was that I was now consciously aware of those walls. And while therapy had helped me to recover feelings and allowed me to make more meaningful connections, it wasn't until Marc entered my life that I gained the courage and strength to open my heart and allow a true, deep connection to develop, fostering intimacy, trust, and the evolution of a relationship.

Having a partner wasn't something I'd planned for or something I even wanted before Marc. *Gay. Relationship. Husband.* Those words were not a part of my vocabulary. They were things that I avoided. I barely knew myself; sex was reserved for strangers and love only happened in movies.

While the possibility that I was gay had gradually taken shape in my head, my views remained sketchy at that time. During the mid-2000s, everybody was talking about acceptance, and the LGBT community was on the cusp of important social change. It seemed easier than ever before for a lot of young people to come out and be who they were, yet I retreated further into the shadows. I couldn't be who I was. I associated "gay" with the man who molested me, and the johns I got paid to screw. The abuse and the hustling were both unbearable sources of shame, and the thought of me being gay, unfortunately, was caught up in that same net.

Meeting Marc changed all of my thinking. I am not saying that my relationship with him came easily, or that there wasn't a huge learning curve, but after discovering a man who so deeply cared for me without wanting something in return, I let go of that shame, and "being gay" wasn't tough anymore. With shame off my shoulders, trust and love didn't seem like mythological creatures anymore. They were real things, things that I was experiencing for the first time since childhood.

After talking to Marc from the hostel balcony in Casco Viejo, and while the hostel parties raged on into the night, I lay in my bunk and opened my Panama travel guide with a smile on my face. In the guide I found a short testimonial from a fellow backpacker about the beauty of the nearby San Blas Islands and how living there, among the native Kuna people, had been a truly humbling experience for him. Impulsively, I made the decision right there and then that I would follow suit. Marc had encouraged this solo adventure for a reason and I would not let him or myself down by turning away from the opportunity that was in front of me. I had to let the past go. I had to catapult myself forward and face the things that made me uncomfortable. I had found true connection with my husband; now, it was time to connect with the rest of the world... and with myself.

In the morning, after a lot of asking around and with tips from locals and other backpackers, I was led to a man, who knew a man, who knew a Kuna family of the Lau clan, who lived on a tiny island in the San Blas Archipelago forty-five miles off the Caribbean coast of Panama. For a meager fee, he would take me there by boat and the family would allow me to live with them for a week in return for a little manual labor and trade of food and comforts from the city. I readily agreed, with almost no information about what I was getting into. My gut was telling me to go.

I hurriedly arranged provisions and trade items, and set out the next morning with an open mind and an open heart. I got aboard the small fishing boat, with the man who knew a man who knew a man, feeling a mix of anxiety and excitement. After a half a day's travel on the open water, the man puttered his boat to a stop on the island.

"*Aqui. Eso es todo,*" he said as he winked and smiled.

"*Muchas gracias.*" I reached over to shake his hand with a crisp twenty-dollar bill between my fingers, the way I had always seen my dad tip people.

I stepped off the boat into the warm shallow blue waters surrounding what I can only describe as an altogether postcard perfect piece of paradise. The hot sun warmed my bare torso like a bear hug. As the water lapped gently against my legs and I gazed forward at this beautiful tiny island spattered with tall coconut palms, my head cleared. All the anxiety, all the anticipation, the fear, my extreme determination to connect...completely gone. Time stood perfectly still in that moment. I knew now. I didn't have to *force* myself to connect to this place or to the people I was about to meet. It was just going to happen.

As time ramped back up to speed, the feeling I experienced was an all-encompassing wholeness. Like I could take on anybody, any-place, and any situation with a clear mind, void of the distractions and pain of my past. It was a confidence that I had never experi-enced before and that I possess to this day.

From out of a palm-thatched hut in the center of the tiny island, two impossibly adorable little Kuna girls came running down the beach to greet me. I flung open my arms wide and they both crashed into me with a hug.

"*¡Hola, chicas!*" I said gently.

"*¡Hola!*" they each yelled back, almost in unison.

The older girl pointed to her younger sister, "*Dendalles,*" and pointed to herself, "*Shrudalles.*"

Then they both pointed at me.

"*Soy Jordan — ¡mucho gusto!*" I said in my shaky Spanish.

They both looked at me with a confused smile and it was then I realized that they didn't know the Spanish language and spoke in their own Kuna dialect. They said a few Kuna words that I didn't understand and finally just grabbed my hand, dragging me back to the hut where I was introduced to the rest of my host family.

Without understanding a word of what was spoken, I felt like I belonged.

I spent the following six days with that wonderful family work-ing, and learning about the island and their culture and how they survived isolated from the mainland. We fished and cooked and helped to repair their shelter. I played with the girls and watched the little one while the mother did the washing. The whole experience had such an immediate and important impact on me, not only because of the beauty of the island or the experience of living without any modern comforts, but because I had successfully and effortlessly connected and integrated with this family, even without the use of language. In those few short days, the Lau family transported me back to the me who had played on the farm in my Osh-Kosh overalls, back to a time where I didn't have to second guess my thoughts and feelings and judge whether they were appropriate or not. The family had unknowingly taught me that I could, in fact, connect and be intimate with others without any ulterior motives or sexual stigma attached. It was a lesson I desperately needed to learn. My eyes were now wide open.

I know first hand how incredibly easy it is to get stuck in "survivor" mode. Until those days on the island, that was where I was. I was married to a man beyond my dreams, living a life I never thought possible, I spent years in recovery with tons of support, yet I still remained the poster boy for "that kid who survived childhood sexual abuse" and had for so long I thought that was all I could be. For years, people told me how moved they were to learn I had survived such a tragic experience.

"You're so brave."

"You are an inspiration to so many."

"I look up to you for the courage you have through all this."

"Congratulations. You beat this."

While I was grateful for the kind words and thoughts, constant praise and affirmations had made me complacent with my life, like

I had already done my part on this planet by just surviving my childhood. It was not a full life, though, because I remained defined by the abuse.

If I had to select just one gift that those islands and those mountains and those jungles gave to me, it is the understanding that there is so much more to me than surviving sexual abuse. It is a huge part of me, sure, but look at me now.

Traveling with an open heart changed my entire outlook on life. I witnessed firsthand that the world is *not* a horrible place waiting to rip me apart, but instead an incredibly beautiful and inviting place that is begging for me to discover it. I moved on from the islands of Panama to explore the continent of South America with my newfound confidence, making connections with so many incredible people and places along the way. I climbed mountains and volcanoes in Chile, bungee jumped off bridges and waterfalls in Ecuador, and got foam-blasted at street parties in Peru.

And, of course, I made peace with that giant fly from the Bolivian jungle.

∴

I am released from the grip of the toxic, sticky tar that comes with sexual abuse. I am truly living now; happy, experiencing, achieving, loving, and on the bullet train back to my 24-carat self.

Jordan Masciangelo has been publicly speaking about overcoming childhood trauma for over seven years, working in support of numerous outreach initiatives including the Ontario Provincial Police, the Canadian Centre for Abuse Awareness, Malesurvivor.org, and All Children Matter. Jordan has been featured on Canadian Broadcasting Corporation Radio, The Oprah Winfrey Show, *Oprah Winfrey Network's* Where Are They Now?, *and End Child Prostitution and*

Trafficking Canada's **Man to Man** *campaign as well as in newspaper and online articles. In 2012, he was honored by the Governor General of Canada with the prestigious Queen Elizabeth II Diamond Jubilee Medal for his contribution, commitment, and ongoing-efforts to the Canadian people and the betterment of his country. Originally from Toronto, Canada, Jordan now resides with his husband and three dogs in sunny Miami, Florida.*

My Red Wedding Dress

Caitlin Heather

I sit down to write but the words are stuck, all stopped up at the back of my throat. The back of my throat is a place I have come to know well over the years as the gatekeeper of my voice. I was silenced when I was seven, my story buried beneath the sands of time and life and denial.

As the grains trickled through the proverbial hourglass, I grew into a woman. Although my story no longer burned at the back of my throat, it was far from forgotten. It made its way down into my belly and into my vagina, and the fire manifested as digestive troubles and painful sex. My throat might as well have been a lead pipe stuffed with rocks, for my voice had all but vanished.

So I wrote poetry, went to therapy, practiced yoga, danced, and joined women's groups. I learned to meditate and commune with the Goddess and the Earth. I even fell in love. And all these things healed me little by little, but still the burning remained, still my poetry was haunted by figures in black and little girls who couldn't scream.

My husband and I have been through the anger and the pain of illness, family burden, and loss. I wanted to be free of the burdens of my past, to be able to have sex with my husband. In the first year of our relationship, I was diagnosed with vulvar vestibulitis, a painful inflammatory condition affecting the vestibule of the vagina. Even on a good day, the pain was too intense to allow sexual penetration. For over five years, we were unable to have what most people consider "sex." Sure, we explored alternatives to penetrative sex, but no matter what people said, no amount of tantric breathing or aligning of our chakras truly fulfilled our yearning for intercourse.

As I began searching for the key to unlock my shackles, one of the first things I did was sign up for voice lessons.

At my first lesson, the teacher struck a note on the piano and asked if I could match it. I opened my mouth, but all that came out were sobs, and I melted into a puddle on the floor. Learning to make sound was one of the most terrifying things I had ever done. But it has changed me. In the past year, I have learned to sing and to speak in front of a group, and I no longer run out of breath just from talking.

With the return of my voice has come an empowered sense of who I am. The burning at the back of my throat has fueled an intense desire to share my story, for it has become clear to me that I cannot transform the trauma and the pain within the silent confines of my body. My story needs breath and freedom. She needs to be witnessed, and she longs to inspire others to heal as well.

A few days before my wedding, I knew I had to confront my family and the part they had played in my story. I asked them to take responsibility, now, for the choices they made when I was a child, and to hear me now as a grown woman asking for their love and their support in carrying the story and moving forward. I explained that it was far too heavy a load to have been placed on the shoulders of a little girl, and as I stood an empowered woman before my wedding altar, it was a burden I was no longer willing to bear alone.

In the days that followed my wedding, I was visited at night by a shadowy figure with red eyes. He told me he was bound to me and that without him I could not be safe. Though shaken by this strange presence, I eventually realized he was nothing more than the years of silence and secrecy woven into the shape of a man. I recognized in my heart and in my mind that I no longer needed him, and with that he was gone.

Since then, things have been different. Mysterious, residual illnesses have begun their retreat from my body, and I have become less and less afraid of the world. I have gone back to school. I've gotten health insurance and proper medical care for the remaining pain in my wildly courageous vagina. I have tracked down the court records from my childhood and uncovered truths I didn't know. I combed through the boxes of old journals in my closet and revisited the writing held hostage amidst the glitter-gel-pen pages of my adolescent self.

This is the moment I have been waiting for: the chance to share my story and set her free.

Today, I grant you freedom, story of mine. Go forth and live on the wings of the breeze, on the breath of the muses from ancient times. I am no longer afraid of being raped or silenced or burned at the stake for speaking my truth. I will keep no more secrets. I will tell no more witch-hunt tales. I am done being a victim!

I am strong and I am whole. I will no longer sit idly by and be violated again and again and again. I will walk on my own two feet; I will dance and I will heal. I will let into the sacred temple of my body all the pleasure I have been denied, and all the pleasure denied to my mother before me and her mother before her.

And what of the fire at the back of my throat? I will sing it out for the world to hear, and I pray it will inspire others who have been silenced as I once was.

When I married, I chose to live my life in the present. I am a free and healthy woman, no longer bound by the past. I marked this passage by getting married in a red dress.

My Red Wedding Dress

In myth, it is the maiden who wears white. She is young, pure, a virgin. She is also often raped. Or at least dragged into the Underworld.

I do not come to this marriage a young, pure virgin. I am neither frightened nor naïve.

I have already lived the stories of violation in my own maidenhood, and I have done too much work, emotionally, psychologically, and spiritually, to bring any remnants of these stories into my marriage.

I do not come to this marriage as a girl, or a victim. I am not marrying for politics, power, money, or escape.

I am a 29-year-old empowered woman, and I choose to marry for love!

I leave behind the stories of fear and abuse, rape and victimhood. These are the stories the women in my family have brought to the altar for generations, and needless to say, they have not found themselves in happy marriages. I, too, inherited and lived these stories, and today I choose to step out of them.

From amidst the dusty pages of the storybooks and family photo albums of my childhood, I emerge, a woman free to make her own choices.

I choose a relationship of health and happiness. My marriage to my beloved will be one of truth and of passion. Of honesty and healing.

Together, we have cried and battled and grieved and yearned. We have held each other in our deepest fears, and also in profound love. It is with all of this that we choose consciously and excitedly to do this together: To continue loving each other and healing ourselves.

I wear red to our wedding to represent our passion and love for each other. The healthy sexual relationship we are seeking and creating. The home and roots we will build together.

In myth, it is the maiden who wears white. She is innocent and sweet, and does not yet know the pleasures of the flesh.

I know with every cell in my body the pleasure and the pain of sex. I am not interested in bringing the stories of rape and abuse from the mythic world, nor from my family, to my wedding.

I am a strong and empowered woman who chooses to be in a healthy relationship with an awesome man!

My red wedding dress is a badge. It says: Look what I've done! Look how much I've healed! Look at the wonderful man I've found! It says, this lineage of abused women stops with me.

Let this marriage be a fanfare of love! A celebration of triumph, and glory yet to come.

Let this marriage be as strong and as bold, as passionate and as sexy, as beautiful and unapologetic as my red dress!

Caitlin Heather lives with her husband and dog in Boulder, Colorado. She is a Spanish-English court interpreter, practicing pagan, and poet.

Afterword

Incidents of harm to our physical and psychosocial selves—particularly patterns of ongoing abuse—cause a common response in humans, which is to "layer up," to wrap ourselves in psychic gauze to cover the wounds inside. This gauze can aid in the healing process, but oftentimes not only covers over wounds but also shrouds our spirits—the very essence of who we are. It is the act of unraveling the protective gauze, of exposing the now-healed wounds, that allows for our true selves to emerge

That's the lesson to take from these 17 stories. Healing is possible. Reclaiming desire is possible. Living fully is possible.

Beyond any commonalities in their histories or emotions, the contributors found joy in writing about their journeys, which was often lonely and rarely linear. For many, writing has provided the opportunity to reflect on how far they have come and take note of their own fortitude. They have honored those who have helped them find their way and have taken another step deeper into their healing. Their vulnerability, tenacity, skill, and substance are palpable and profound.

Many contributors voiced that they didn't necessarily or always feel that they had fully moved "beyond" surviving. In the process of writing, many suffered waves of uncertainty that challenged their initial confidence: "Who am I to tell anyone what the process is?" "Some days I'm there, other days I'm not." "This had better not be all there is because I want more."

In spite of their concerns, we believe that they have moved beyond survival mode. All of these writers continue to reach new heights in their recovery. They find themselves with more freedom and less protective covering. They feel more comfortable and confident as sexual beings. They have discovered the happy pleasure of making out like a virgin, unencumbered by the past.

We observed that the dread of telling one's story could sit side by side with the energy and desire to share it. For some, the anguish of opening up old wounds or facing in print what they would rather forget was hard to overcome. For various reasons, a few people made the decision to withdraw from the project. Whether or not they are in this book, they are well on their way in their own journey.

We are most grateful to our contributors. We are honored to know them. They show us that being someone who has experienced and survived sexual trauma is not a limitation. They now lead lives with a wholeness of spirit along with a spunk that propels them forward to everything that is possible. Their courage and resilience is a guiding light. We admire and adore them all. We deeply and especially thank them for trusting us with their stories.

This book is an invitation for more people to tell the story of how they have triumphed, how they have come to a point where they are no longer defined by the trauma.

For those starting their journey toward reclaiming a healthy sexuality, there are many excellent resources, workbooks, tools, and advocates available. In many countries there are national and local organizations that address sexual violence and support those in need. We hope you find ones that lift you and provide optimism.

We sincerely wish that everyone finds the freedom to make out like a virgin, and, if they choose, have earth-shaking, sky-raising, lusty sex, desire, and intimacy. Because it's not just a kiss. A kiss is sensuous and expansive and flush with anticipation; it is the start of an exciting and natural phenomenon.

Catriona & Cathy

The Editors

CATRIONA MCHARDY

Catriona McHardy has spent her life studying human sexuality and formally held a career promoting healthy expressions of sexuality, individually and culturally. In 32 years at Planned Parenthood of Northern New England, she rose from health care associate to longtime Vice President for Education and Training. She led a team of "sexperts" who provided sexuality education and training to professionals, teens, and parents regionally, nationally, and internationally, including Africa and Russia.

Catriona is currently a consultant and trainer on issues pertaining to sexual expression and sex positive culture. She is also a faculty member at Community College of Vermont, where she teaches courses in communication, race, ethnicity, class and gender, and human sexuality. She has served as national co-chair of the Association of Planned Parenthood Leaders in Education and served her community on the boards of the Women's Crisis Center in Brattleboro, Vermont and Outright Vermont, as well as the Governor's Task Force on Gender Bias in the Courts and the Vermont Task Force on Teen Pregnancy.

CATHY PLOURDE

Cathy's plays on coping with eating disorders (*The Thin Line*) and engaging bystanders in interrupting violence (*You the Man*) have been presented across the US and have been culturally translated for use in Australia. She has presented and published nationally and internationally on theatre and arts for social change, wellness, education, and community building, and has received commissions and artist residencies from numerous organizations to develop works addressing these issues.

As founder and director of Add Verb Productions she raised over a million dollars in grant awards, private donations, and performance fees to promote this work, including the award-winning performance and activism anthologies (*Out & Allied*, vol. 1 and 2) for LGBTQ youth and their allies. She was a long-standing Honorary Artist in Residence at the University of Southern Maine, served as a founding member of Boys to Men Maine and the Pride Youth Theatre Alliance, and taught Integrated Health Sciences at the University of New England.

Acknowledgements

We feel so lucky to know each of the people on the team of supporters surrounding this book. This circle reaches back decades and includes people who have grounded us in the field of sex education and the in the prevention of and intervention in sexual and domestic violence.

There are two particular women without whom we could not have done this. They believed in our abilities and our vision, and generously added their skills into the sauce:

Dee Steffan, we are indebted to you for your extraordinary writing and copyediting expertise, your brilliant ability to clarify and see where we wanted to go at times before we did. For the countless hours you gave us as a sounding board, publicist, and voice of reason, thank you.

Kara, it would not have been possible without your daily support.

Tavia Gilbert, Portlyn Media, and Animal Mineral Press, thank you for your 30,000 foot view with hawk-eyed precision and generous flexibility as the three of us sat around the table. We are grateful for the opportunity.

Sue William Silverman, we could not have found a more gracious and generous writer for the foreword.

To our advance readers who helped push this out in the world, thank you for expanding the circle of people who can give more light to the possibilities.

Special thanks to our slew of friends who listened and advised and cared for the outcome of this project.

And thanks to the creatives: kd diamond, for your lovely cover design; Spencer Worthley, for assisting so steadily in building our space online; David Camlin, who offered not only video expertise, but as ever, great kindness and friendship; and Jen and Rachel of Over the River, your guidance remains invaluable.

CPSIA information can be obtained at www.ICGtesting.com
Printed in the USA
BVOW02s1209210816

459574BV00003B/4/P

The common thread through this collection of moving essays is courage, hope and inspiration. What a gift to anyone recovering from sexual trauma or anyone wanting to accompany them on their journeys to recovery and fulfillment.

David Walsh, Ph.D. Psychologist and author of
Why Do They Act That Way? A Survival Guide to the Adolescent Brain for You and Your Teen

Though of different countries, races, genders, orientations, backgrounds, and experiences, their tales weave together a tapestry of courage, strength, resourcefulness, resilience, and hope.

Luca Maurer, co-author of *The Teaching Transgender Toolkit*

Immensely helpful to those who call themselves victims and those who call themselves survivors and those readers looking for a more complex understanding of sexuality after trauma, growth, recovery, and healing.

Sharon Lamb, Ed.D., Ph.D., ABPP, author of *Packaging Girlhood* and *Sex, Therapy, and Kids*

A lifeline to anyone who is raped or sexually abused.

Carol Ness, editor, writer, UC Berkeley

There is a way through sexual trauma:
Forever changed, yes, but not forever damaged.

Jacqueline S. Weinstock, Ph.D., Human Development & Family Studies, University of Vermont

Through these powerful, beautiful stories we recognize that life is complicated, messy, painful, and damaging. But like the phoenix from the ashes, healing hope, driving passions, and a deep love of self can be born amidst the rubble.

Auburn L. Watersong, Associate Director of Public Policy,
Vermont Network Against Domestic and Sexual Violence and Episcopal Priest

This collection fills a gap in available literature about survivorship and healing and is a gift for those of us working alongside survivors and those of us who are survivors ourselves. These are stories of survivors coming back into their spontaneity, their vivaciousness, and their desire.

Jen Friedlander, Washington Coalition of Sexual Assault Programs

$16.99
ISBN 978-1-944568-00-9
51699>

AVAILABLE IN AUDIO, EBOOK, AND PRINT
FROM ANIMALMINERALPRESS.COM

MAKING OUT LIKE A
LIKE A
VIRGIN

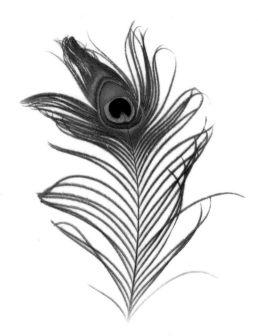

Sex, Desire & Intimacy
After Sexual Trauma

EDITED BY
CATRIONA MCHARDY AND CATHY PLOURDE